Clinical Essays in Obstetrics and Gynaecology for MRCOG Part II
(And Other Postgraduate Exams)

Seema Sharma
MRCOG, MD, DGO
Consultant Obstetrician and Gynecologist
New Delhi
drseemagyn@hotmail.com

Mala Arora
FRCOG (UK), FICOG, FICMCH, DA (UK)
Chairperson FOGSI Quiz Committee
Faridabad
malanarinder@yahoo.com

Foreword

Anthony Hollingworth

JAYPEE BROTHERS
MEDICAL PUBLISHERS (P) LTD.
NEW DELHI

Published by

Jitendar P Vij

Jaypee Brothers Medical Publishers (P) Ltd

B-3, EMCA House, 23/23B Ansari Road, Daryaganj, **New Delhi** 110 002, India

Phones: +91-11-23272143, +91-11-23272703, +91-11-23282021, +91-11-23245672

Rel: 32558559   Fax: +91-11-23276490, +91-11-23245683

e-mail: jaypee@jaypeebrothers.com   Visit our website: www.jaypeebrothers.com

Branches

- 2/B, Akruti Society, Jodhpur Gam Road Satellite, **Ahmedabad** 380 015
  Phones: +91-079-26926233,   Rel: +91-079-32988717,   Fax: +91-079-26927094
  e-mail: jpamdvd@rediffmail.com

- 202 Batavia Chambers, 8 Kumara Krupa Road, Kumara Park East, **Bangalore** 560 001
  Phones: +91-80-22285971, +91-80-22382956,   Rel: +91-80-32714073
  Fax: +91-80-22281761   e-mail: jaypeemedpubbgl@eth.net

- 282 IIIrd Floor, Khaleel Shirazi Estate, Fountain Plaza, Pantheon Road, **Chennai** 600 008
  Phones: +91-44-28193265, +91-44-28194897,   Rel: +91-44-32972089
  Fax: +91-44-28193231   e-mail: jpchen@eth.net

- 4-2-1067/1-3, 1st Floor, Balaji Building, Ramkote Cross Road, **Hyderabad** 500 095
  Phones: +91-40-66610020, +91-40-24758498,   Rel:+91-40-32940929
  Fax:+91-40-24758499,   e-mail: jpmedpub@rediffmail.com

- No. 41/3098, B & B1, Kuruvi Building, St. Vincent Road, **Kochi** 682 018, Kerala
  Phones: +91-0484-4036109, +91-0484-2395739, +91-0484-2395740
  e-mail: jaypeekochi@rediffmail.com

- 1-A Indian Mirror Street, Wellington Square, **Kolkata** 700 013
  Phones: +91-33-22451926, +91-33-22276404, +91-33-22276415,   Rel: +91-33-32901926
  Fax: +91-33-22456075,   e-mail: jpbcal@dataone.in

- 106 Amit Industrial Estate, 61 Dr SS Rao Road, Near MGM Hospital, Parel, **Mumbai** 400 012
  Phones: +91-22-24124863, +91-22-24104532,   Rel: +91-22-32926896
  Fax: +91-22-24160828,   e-mail: jpmedpub@bom7.vsnl.net.in

- "KAMALPUSHPA" 38, Reshimbag, Opp. Mohota Science College, Umred Road, **Nagpur** 440 009 (MS)
  Phones: Rel: 3245220,   Fax: 0712-2704275   e-mail: jaypeenagpur@dataone.in

Clinical Essays in Obstetrics and Gynaecology for MRCOG Part II (And Other Postgraduate Exams)

This book has been published in good faith that the material provided by authors is original. Every effort has been made to ensure accuracy of material, but the publisher, printer or editor will not be held responsible for any inadvertent error(s). In case of any dispute, all legal matters would be settled under Delhi jurisdiction only.

First Edition: **2007**

ISBN 81-8448-007-5

Typeset at JPBMP typesetting unit

Printed at   Rajkamal Electric Press, G.T.Karnal Road, Industrial Area, Delhi-33

Obste Gynecology

MCQs

(And Othe Exams)

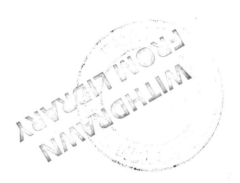

Dedicated to

*All the students sitting
postgraduate examinations*

Foreword

Preparing for any examination can be a daunting task. It is paramount when studying for the MRCOG Part 2 examination that no area of the curriculum be omitted. This book covers a wide range of topics and should prove invaluable in the preparation for the written part of the examination. Technique and time management in answering the written papers are essential and the examples in this book will help give a systematic approach to the short essay questions.

Anthony Hollingworth
MB ChB (Manchester) MBA (Keele)
PhD (London) FRCS (Ed), FRCOG
Consultant in O & G
Whipps Cross University Hospital Trust
London

Preface

While I was preparing for my MRCOG 2 written examination, I felt the need to have a comprehensive book on essay writing skills. Very few were available in India then. Hence, the present attempt is made. Beside MRCOG, postgraduate students appearing for Diploma, National Board and MD examinations may find it useful.

Though the field of obstetrics and gynecology is vast, yet the choice of questions has been narrowed down to topics which the students find difficult to answer. To keep the essays updated, most of the recent advances have been referred to while writing the book.

Important points for general understanding and MCQs have been incorporated in the form of notes at the end of each essay. We have tried to make this book handy and readable. Keeping in view the changed format of the MRCOG 2 theory exam, a few questions towards the end have been answered accordingly. We sincerely hope that readers will find it useful and pass their examination in the first attempt.

This book has been designed for students and suggestions to improve the structure, content or layout is welcome.

Seema Sharma
drseemagyn@hotmail.com

Acknowledgements

Mr Anthony Hollingworth has been my teacher and provided clarity of thought and content all along. I thank him for supporting us for this project.

My children, Hriday and Niyati and my husband Sandeep have all been very understanding, generous and patient with me all this while. Without their help this book would have never seen the light of the day.

Contents

Part 2: Gynecology

TIPS for Preparing the Part 2 MRCOG Exam

This is a very comprehensive exam and one needs to be through and updated. Enroll for the trainees register and visit the RCOG website frequently. Read all the guidelines and statements issued by the college, including the NICE, FFPRC guidelines, and CEMACH reports.

Read as many SAQ books as possible. It is best to attempt at least one question per day in stipulated time but if that is not possible at least go through the text in your free time. It familiarizes the student with the essay techniques and decreases the possibility of encountering the unknown at the time of final examination.

Make your own list of common percentages from the guidelines and other text on the RCOG website. List of autosomal dominant and recessive conditions, survival at key gestational ages, various stages of malignancies with their survival can be similarly prepared. Keep this list handy and refer to it frequently so they can be used in essay questions to support your arguments and in Multiple Choice Questions.

It helps to keep cool. Practice some kind of meditation, exercise or deep breathing skills.

At least two weeks prior to the examination date, set your circadian rhythms according to the examination timetable for optimal performance. Practice the essays, MCQs and EMQs as if you are in the actual examination situation.

Learn to incorporate certain terms in your essays, the politically correct words as they say;

- Multidisciplinary treatment,
- Information leaflets/written information to the women
- Additional counseling whenever she requires.
- Informed decision by the woman, sympathetic and nonjudgmental attitude
- Anti-D wherever applicable, in a nonsensitized rhesus negative woman,
- Develop hospital audits or local protocols,
- Refer to specialist care or tertiary set up, involve support groups.
- Do not forget to add that some women with a given condition may be normal and require only reassurance.
- Clear documentation of counseling/procedure/woman's wishes in the case files.

I would like to recommend that the student just scribbles these phrases onto the rough work sheet and add whatever required in each essay according to the situation. This would definitely add a few marks and thus be invaluable to the borderline candidates.

TIPS TO FORMULATE THE ESSAY ANSWER:

- Read the question 2-3 times and establish what is being asked. Do not be in a hurry to show your expertise on that topic. Underline the key words if you like. Remember that these details especially the ones about age, parity and lifestyle are there for a particular reason and formulate your answers accordingly. Pain abdomen in early first trimester, i.e. 6-8 weeks is more likely to be ectopic; 24 weeks is the legal time of viability; 34 weeks, after which antenatal steroids are no longer recommended; 38 weeks, maturity; 41 weeks at which induction is beneficial. Ask yourself why this information is there and what happens at this time or to a woman of this parity.

- Think straight. They are asking you about everyday things that you have done and experienced before. Think of all possible angles—related to patient, her relatives, and medical personnel in that particular situation. Start with simple, straight forward physiological things first. Do not doubt the intentions of the examiners. Usually there are no hidden complexities in the question. If the question asks about management of premature rupture of membranes, do not waste space by trying to establish if leaking is actually present or not. Assume it is the correct diagnosis. If you feel very strongly about establishing the diagnosis mention a line that you would like to reconfirm/establish the diagnosis/presentation.

- Plan your answer and jot down important points that you will incorporate. Never leave a question unanswered. Jot down whatever point comes to your mind regarding that. You are likely to score a few marks that can make the difference. One essay is likely to be out of the blue but DO NOT PANIC. It is tough for everyone. Think how you can maximize your scores. Even while reading the questions, a fleeting vague thought comes in your mind, quickly scribble on the rough sheet. You may forget it later in the exam anxiety.

  One can ask for extra rough sheets but not the actual answering sheet.

- Write in short simple sentences with legible handwriting. You may highlight important points. Avoid repetitions in various forms. It utilizes space without adding on marks. Do not get sidetracked while writing and start adding subpoints to the highlighted point. It is important to give the global picture and incorporate all the important points before one runs out of space. Usually there is no need for introduction and conclusion in the essay plan unless it stresses a point not otherwise covered in the essay.

- The space provided for answering the essays is limited. Hence, memorize some space saver phrases like –
  - Medical optimization prior to surgery,
  - A risk and need assessment at booking with individualized flexible care plan
  - Woman's wishes and viewpoints etc.
- There are certain critical phrases in the question which are useful templates according to which the essay structure should be built.

Critical appraisal/evaluation
Describe available options and discuss pros and cons.
Justify your choice on the basis of evidence. Assess the value of the chosen option.

Counseling
Describe the risks and benefits. Describe and justify your management in the light of other available options and risks. Informed consent from the patient is essential.

Diagnosis
History, examination and appropriate investigations.

Management
Diagnosis, medical, surgical and supportive treatment.

Plan of care for a pregnant woman
Starts with antenatal assessment, fetal and maternal monitoring with management of condition.
Intrapartum management; including mode of delivery.
Postpartum care; including advice on breastfeeding, contraception and preconception counseling for next pregnancy; if applicable.

Usefulness as a screening test
Emphasize that screening test is not diagnostic. What are the criteria for screen positives, risks and potential benefits of diagnosis. Are treatment options available if diagnosis is confirmed and are they acceptable to the patient?

- Revise your answer towards the end when you are in a more balanced state of mind.

The new format of MRCOG part 2 written examination
(Effective from the examination sitting of 5 September 2006 onwards)
There are essentially three main components for the written examination;
Short answer questions: There is an essay paper each for obstetrics and gynecology, each with four short essays; instead of five. The time duration allowed to complete each paper has been reduced from two hours to one hour forty five minutes, so candidates have twenty six minutes to answer each question. According to the new format; there are two or three components for each essay, representing different aspects of that condition. There is a specific space to answer each component and one cannot exceed that space or use space meant for answering other components. An example is given below for clarification:

Question: You are the SpR on emergency duty and you have just been informed that the SHO on duty has created a uterine perforation while performing an MTP.
a. What is your initial assessment of the case on reaching the theater?
   Three blank lines given to complete the answer.
b. How will you manage the case in theater?
   Five to six blank lines to complete the answer.
c. What will be your postoperative management of the case?
   Four to five blank lines to answer the question.
   Separate marks will be allotted to each component. Clearly one needs clarity of thought and be able to put specific information within the space provided. It comprises 60% of the total marks for written assessment.
   Though most of the work for this book was finished before the format for the written examination changed; we have tried to incorporate a few essays in the new format towards the end of the book.

Multiple Choice Questions: This section has been retained as in the previous years except remained. These comprise 25% of the total value. There is a lead statement followed by a few responses > each of them have to be marked true or false > there is no negative marking for the incorrect responses.

Extended Matching Questions (EMQs): Introduction of EMQs is the major change in the new format. They comprise 15% of the total value of marks for the written examination. Each EMQ consists of a lead—in statement, and then a list of one to five questions (each numbered to match the answer sheet) and an option list. Each option list may be used for just one question or a number of questions. From the list each option may be used once < more than once or none at all >> The candidates will be provided with a question booklet and an answersheet, which they have to fill by darkening the lozenges with a HB pencil only. The candidates must select the single best option and mark it. No marks are awarded if more than one box is marked. There is no negative marking for incorrect responses and each EMQ paper has a standard setting by the RCOG with a varying passmark each time. This sheet is later on read and marked by a computer.

The **timetable** for the written paper looks something like this;

Short answer questions Paper 1; 15 minute break

MCQ Paper; 45 minute lunch break

EMQ Paper; 15 minute break

Short Answer Questions Paper 2

Length and question numbers of papers

Short Answers	2 Papers, each 1 hour forty five min.	8 questions overall
EMQ Paper	1 hour	40 questions
MCQ Paper	1 hour thirty minutes	225 questions

PART 1
Obstetrics

PAPER 1

1. A second gravida attends your clinic at 36 weeks gestation to discuss the pros and cons of her delivery. Her first delivery was by cesarean section and she is medically fit.

2. A woman of Asian origin residing in UK wants to travel to India for vacation. She is currently 24 weeks pregnant. Outline the advice you will give her.

3. A 30-year-old woman has recently been diagnosed as having Systemic Lupus Erythematosus (SLE). She wishes to start her family and comes to you for advice. Briefly outline her preconception and prenatal management.

4. You are the Obstetrics and Gynecology Senior Registrar (SpR$_3$) in a unit delivering 4,500 women per year. It is mid-afternoon, and suddenly the emergency buzzer goes off in Room 6 and an anxious midwife puts her head out of the door and shouts "patient hemorrhaging". Describe your actions in detail in the next 30 min.

1. **A second gravida attends your clinic at 36 weeks gestation to discuss the pros and cons of her delivery. Her first delivery was by cesarean section and she is medically fit.**

The decision about mode of birth should take into consideration maternal preferences and priorities. She must be involved in decision making but her request on its own is not an automatic indication for planned cesarean section. Specific reasons for her request should be explored, discussed and recorded.

The success rates for vaginal birth after cesarean section **(VBAC)** vary from 60-80% and are altered by the indication of first section. She should be informed about the overall risks and benefits of cesarean section:

With c-section there is less perineal pain along with decreased incidence of urinary incontinence (after 3 months) and uterovaginal prolapse. Risk of intrapartum infant death is 10 times lower in planned c-section. Neonatal morbidity is decreased in breech presentations and noncephalic first twin pregnancies.

There is an increased incidence of abdominal pain, bladder and ureteric injury, need for further surgery (laprotomy, dilatation and curettage or hysterectomy), admission to intensive care unit, thromboembolic disease, longer hospital stay hospital readmissions and maternal death. If performed before 38 completed weeks, it can increase neonatal respiratory morbidity (Transient tachypnoea of the newborn). The implications for future pregnancies include an increased incidence of having no more children, placenta previa, morbidly adherent placenta, uterine rupture before labor and ante partum still birth.

There is no effect of mode of delivery on blood loss > 1000 ml, wound infection (endometritis), genital tract injury, fecal incontinence, backpain, postnatal depression and dyspareunia. No difference in the incidence of neonatal mortality (excluding breech), intracranial hemorrhage, brachial plexus injury and cerebral palsy has been found.

Uterine rupture is a rare complication but the risk of dehiscence is higher with VBAC. A previous classical CS or an unknown uterine scar is a contraindication to VBAC due to higher incidence (4 times) of scar dehiscence.

Once a cesarean section, always a hospital delivery and there is no place for domiciliary management of such pregnancies. If the women is not satisfied and insists for an electric C-section, another senior consultant should also be involved in decision making and subsequent counseling.

2. **An apparently healthy woman of Asian origin residing in UK wants to travel to India for vacation. She is currently 24 weeks pregnant. Outline the advice you will give her.**

The journey from UK to India is a long haul flight (> 3 hours duration). In the absence of major medical and obstetric complications, air travel is quite safe and she should be reassured about the same.

Advise her to take a *medical travel insurance* which covers overseas antenatal checkups, delivery and neonatal expenses should the situation arise. She should check with the concerned airline about return flight restrictions. Most airlines do not allow a woman passenger on board with > 34 weeks pregnancy. Some may require a doctor's letter to confirm fitness to travel.

Vaccinations recommended for travel to India are—Hepatitis A, Polio (prefer inject able instead of oral vaccine); tetanus toxoid, typhoid, and tuberculosis (BCG). Optional vaccines are Meningococcal Meningitis (Delhi, Nepal, Pakistan) and post exposure Rabies vaccine (if required).

India is endemic for **malaria** and she should take precautions to avoid mosquito bite. Long sleeved dresses should be worn; coils, candles, insect repellents and mosquito nets should be used for the same. Chloroquine 300 g weekly can be safely started one week before travel till 4 weeks on return. Alternatively, Mefloquine 250 mg weekly for Chloroquine resistant areas can be prescribed.

There is no danger from X-ray security devices at the airport. She should preferably opt for aisle seat instead of window as it gives more leg room and facilitates taking short walks in aircraft.

Pyridoxine can be taken for **travel sickness**. Since pregnancy increases her chances of **thromboembolism** she needs to take plenty of nonalcoholic beverages; maintain lower limb mobility and do regular deep breathing while on board. She should wear below knee Thromboembolic deterrent (TED) stockings.

For Woman at high risk for thromboembolism (obesity, thrombophilia, SLE etc) consider low dose aspirin starting 3 days before and on the day of journey. Alternatively LMWH (dalteparin-5000IU) single dose on the day of travel and one day after, suffices to counter the higher risk of Thrombosis associated with air travel.

On reaching the destination, precautions should be taken for **food and water safety**. She should avoid raw food and drink safe water (boiled, or bottled). Taking frequent small meals and avoiding caffeine can help to overcome jet lag quickly. She should take care to prevent dehydration and heat strokes.

Provide her with RCOG published patient **information leaflet**— "Traveling in pregnancy" for any further clarifications.

Note: *Women with placenta previa, sickle cell disease, severe hypertension and severe anemia (<8.5%) should be advised against air travel during pregnancy. Women with previous history of preterm labor and placental abruption, multiple pregnancies, recent bleeding or any invasive procedure should be informed clearly about unexpected obstetric emergencies and lack of medical facilities on board.*

3. **A 30-year-old woman has recently been diagnosed as having Systemic Lupus Erythematosis (SLE). She wishes to start her family and comes to you for advice. Briefly outline her pre-conception and prenatal management.**

SLE is a systemic connective tissue disease characterized by periods of disease activity (flares) and remissions. Severe disease flare may be potentially life threatening and fetomaternal outcome is improved if disease is in remission for at least 6 months prior to conception.

Knowledge of the antiphospholipid, anti Ro, anti La antibody, renal and blood pressure status and immunosuppressive therapy allows prediction of the risks to the women and her fetus. 6% women have associated autoimmune disorders and appropriate investigations should be advised for the same.

Some drug therapies are teratogenic and fetotoxic. Appropriate dose adjustments to achieve optimal control should be established. If possible discontinue Methotrexate, Mycophenolate and cyclophosphamide for at least 3 months prior to conception due to long half-life and possible teratogenicity.

Counsel patient regarding increased potential for SLE flares, spontaneous miscarriage, intrauterine growth restriction during pregnancy, pre-eclampsia, preterm delivery and fetal death. In the absence of renal disease the pregnancy outcome is similar to that of general population.

Prescribe effective contraception till medical optimization is achieved.

General advice regarding rubella status, folic acid supplementation and avoidance of smoking should be imparted.

Antenatal care should be undertaken by a multidisciplinary team, in a tertiary care setting with experienced staff. Encourage early booking with a first trimester scan to establish accurate dates.

Baseline investigations include complete blood counts (anemia and thrombocytopenia), renal functions, double stranded DNA (ds DNA), anti Ro, La, Smith and anticardiolipin antibodies and lupus anticoagulant, urinalysis for proteinuria and red cell casts. If she has known renal disease, 24 hours urinary proteins and creatinine clearance should be done. Repeat appropriate investigations at 4 weekly intervals.

Maintain antenatal schedule of 2 weeks till the second trimester and weekly thereafter.

Watch for signs and symptoms of SLE flare. These include hypertension, hematuria with rising proteinuria and red cell casts on urinalysis. Investigation show increasing titers of ds DNA, serum creatinine, normal C reactive protein (CRP) and falling complement levels (C3, C4) with thrombocytopenia.

Fetal surveillance with regular growth scans after 20 weeks, Doppler velocimetry at 24 weeks and regularly thereafter to detect fetal growth restriction at the earliest should be undertaken. If mother has positive anti Ro, anti La antibodies, fetal echocardiography should be done at 22 weeks to detect congenital heart block in fetus. Fetal P-R interval measurements, if available can detect first degree heart block.

Low dose aspirin therapy and LMWH (low molecular weight heparin) should be considered if antiphospholipid antibodies are positive. Dexamethasone, salbutamol or digoxin therapy may be judiciously used to revert 2nd degree heart blocks to first and if hydrops fetalis develops.

Glucocorticoids (Prednisolone) can be safely used during pregnancy and to manage flares. Non Steroidal Anti Inflammatory drugs (NSAIDs) particularly Cox -2 selective inhibitors, should be avoided after second trimester. Azathioprim and hydroxychloroquine are the second line therapy and may be continued throughout pregnancy. Methotrexate and cyclosporine are third line therapy. Severe flares may require pulsed methyl prednisolone therapy. Avoid antimalarials and full dose NSAIDs. Hypertension is controlled with methyldopa, with nifedipine or hydralazine as second line drugs.

Deliver at term in absence of complications; avoid postdates. Notify pediatrician and anesthetist at the time of delivery. Steroid boluses may be required at delivery for patients on chronic steroid therapy.

The risk of neonatal lupus is increased if a previous child has been affected but is not related to the severity of maternal disease.

4. **You are the Obstetrics and Gynecology Senior Registrar (Specialist Registrar Year 3) in a unit delivering 4,500 women per year. It is mid-afternoon, and suddenly the emergency buzzer goes off in Room 6 and an anxious midwife puts her head out of the door and shouts "patient hemorrhaging". Describe your actions in detail in the next 30 min.**

Note: If there is a question on Antepartum, postpartum hemorrhage or collapse, the initial management is ABC i.e. A-airway, B-breathing, C-circulation, till patient is stable. Always call for adequate help in emergencies and as part of risk management.

Note: Documentation must be meticulously completed at the earliest possible opportunity.

Ask someone at the reception desk/nurses station to put out an emergency call to the duty Anesthetic registrar, Operating Department Assistant (ODA), and obstetric SHO if not present. Ask obstetric nursing officer to arrange extra staff and the most easily available experienced midwife for room 6. The person concerned will then inform blood bank technician and hematologist about the situation along with the details of the patient. Porters should be summoned to maternity unit for carrying the samples.

Consultant hematologist and obstetrician should be informed of the clinical situation.

Theater should be informed for a possible intervention.

Go to Room 6, quickly find out the patient's name and rapidly introduce yourself in a calm confident manner.

Put a hand on the mother's abdomen to palpate the uterus and ascertain its tone and size, whilst simultaneously "rubbing up" a contraction.

Ask the staff midwife for baseline vitals i.e. pulse, BP and a rapid summary of what has happened so far, including whether or not the placenta is delivered and is complete or not. Make a visual impression about the estimated blood loss.

Give the mother an intramuscular injection of Syntometrine if not hypertensive.

Make an assessment of the mother's cardiovascular state, particularly her pulse rate, and lower the upper part of her bed so that she is lying horizontally. Assign one nurse solely for record keeping; patient's vital signs, urine out put, amount and type of all fluids the patient receives, dosage and type of drugs given.

Insert two large size intravenous cannulae, (preferably 14 gauge) and take 20 ml blood samples from the mother for full blood count, clotting studies and cross matching, and order at least 6 units of blood. Connect an infusion of Hemaccel solution in one and Hartmann's solution in the other line.

Give the mother oxygen to breathe via a face mask, and put a warming blanket over mother's abdomen. Give the staff midwife a Foley catheter to insert into the mother's bladder and connect to a drainage bag.

If placenta and membranes are undelivered, make a further attempt at controlled cord traction and if unsuccessful proceed to manual removal in theater.

If bleeding still continues and uterus is relaxed, commence syntocinon infusion with 10 units' syntocinon. $PGF_{2\alpha}$ (.5-1 mg) can be given straight into uterine muscle, provided she is not asthmatic. Examine the placenta for completeness. Give further bolus of oxytocin if required.

Rule out trauma to vulva, vagina and cervix if uterus remains contracted and bleeding continues.

If bleeding continues, she may need to be taken to theater to explore the uterus for any retained products of conception, trauma or inversion. Apply bimanual compression till anesthesia is administered. Four units of whole blood, 2 units fresh frozen plasma and one unit factor VIII should be ready in the theater.

Exclude coagulation disorder by the preliminary results. Ensure that patient remains hemodynamically stable, replace lost blood and clotting factors. Consider CVP monitoring.

Uterine packing or balloon tamponade can be tried before shifting the patient to theater for further exploration.

Explain patient's condition and the possibility of embolisation/internal iliac ligation/hysterectomy to the attendant.

PAPER 2

1. An 18-year-old woman reveals at her booking visit that she smokes 20-25 cigarettes a day and sniffs cocaine occasionally. She is currently 11 weeks pregnant. How will you manage her pregnancy?

2. A nulliparous woman presents at 36 weeks in casualty with rupture of membranes. Vaginal swab shows growth of group B Streptococcus. How does this information alter your management?

3. A 35-year-old primigravida has been referred to you because her routine anomaly scan at 20 weeks has shown presence of single choroid plexus cyst. Highlight the major issues involved in counseling.

4. 33-year-old primigravida presents at 16 weeks for her first visit. She has a body weight of 140 kg and a body mass index of 40. She has no other apparent risk factor. What problems will you anticipate and counsel for her?

1. **An 18-year-old woman reveals at her booking visit that she smokes 20-25 cigarettes a day and sniffs cocaine occasionally. She is currently 11 weeks pregnant. How will you manage her pregnancy?**

Obtain careful and detailed smoking and drug history, including alcohol consumption. Encourage to maintain drug diary. Maternal and fetal risks depend on the amount and frequency of drug use.

Risks associated with heavy smoking should be told to the woman in clear language. These include miscarriage (more by 25%), placental abruption, placental insufficiency, higher incidence of extrauterine pregnancies, preterm delivery and placenta previa. Risk increases with the number of cigarettes smoked per day so reducing smoking is better than not, but is not as good as stopping. Stopping smoking now will improve pregnancy outcome. Repeated encouragement increases the chances of success and reduces relapse.

Incidence of low birth weight infants, (100-300 g less than average), intrauterine death, neonatal death (one third increase) and sudden infant death syndrome (SIDS) is increased. There are higher chances of neuro developmental impairment in children. The harmful effects far outweigh the slight protective effect against development of pre-eclampsia.

Cocaine abuse compounds the effect on fetus and increases the chances of vascular problems like thrombosis and abruption.

Multidisciplinary approach should be adopted. ENT referral if rhinitis is evident. There is no substitute drug available to help with stabilization in pregnancy.

Confirm dates with a first trimester scan. Rule out anomalies at 20 weeks. Take a high vaginal swab to screen for anaerobic vaginosis. Offer Hepatitis B, hepatitis C and HIV screen. Involve a genitourinary physician if any of the above positive. Sexually transmitted diseases should be screened depending on lifestyle adopted by her to fund the habits. Give adequate iron, vitamin and dietary supplements to prevent malnutrition.

Serial growth scans every 3 weeks after 24 weeks, with Doppler velocimetry if required, to monitor fetal growth.

Plan a meeting at around 32 weeks with the woman, her partner, social and health visitor and community drug team leader to discuss the needs of the woman and her baby. Social, financial, and housing needs along with child protection issues should be discussed.

She should be told not to smoke once contractions have started. There is higher requirement for opiates during labor due to tolerance. She may become violent due to pain causing injury to medical staff. Should general anesthesia be required, she is at high risk for respiratory complications.

Adopt continuous electronic fetal monitoring during labor. Notify Pediatrician to attend delivery. Watch for signs of withdrawal in baby. Baby is at risk of injury due to neglect and vertical transmission of diseases. Attending staff should maintain sympathetic and nonjudgemental attitude and follow Universal precautions at all times.

Notify general practitioner, community and social worker and all people involved in her care at the time of discharge.

Discuss contraception before sending her home.

Note: Pregnant woman are less liable to quit smoking and only one in four stop voluntarily. Most intervention protocols have minimal success.

2. **A nulliparous woman presents at 36 weeks in casualty with rupture of membranes. Vaginal swab shows growth of group B Streptococcus. How does this information alter your management?**

Note: GBS is facultative anaerobic gram positive cocci and can be grown on non selective media. It can be recovered from vagina or cervix in up to 25% of pregnant women at some point during gestation. In majority it is innocuous to mother and baby but in 1/1000 deliveries it causes overwhelming neonatal infection which can be fatal or permanently disabling. History of previous pregnancy affected by GBS is an important risk factor.

Vaginal colonization with group B streptococcus (GBS) is associated with premature rupture of membranes and preterm delivery beyond 32 weeks. There are higher chances of intraamniotic infections, postpartum endometritis, and puerperal septicemia. It is recognized as one of the leading causes of septicemia and meningitis in the first 2 months of life in neonates. Hence she should be offered admission in the hospital and standard labor ward protocol followed to administer tests of maternal and fetal well being.

Delivery at <37 weeks, duration of rupture of membranes = 18 h, and intrapartum fever ≥ 38.0°C are risk factors for development of neonatal GBS.

There is a controversy about preventive strategies and the risks of neonatal GBS infection must be balanced against mother's wishes and the adverse reactions to antibiotics, especially in women with less than 2 risk factors.

A per vaginal examination, should be done to check cervical dilatation and presenting part. Antibiotic chemoprophylaxis for GBS is unnecessary unless she is in established labor. Expectant management may be adopted in such cases in accordance to mother's wishes.

If labor is established or she has ≥ 2 risk factors, chemoprophylaxis should be administered as soon as possible after onset of labor and at least 2 h before delivery. Recommended prophylaxis regimens are:

- Penicillin G 5 mU intravenously, followed by 2.5 mU I.V. every 4 h, or
- Ampicillin 3 g I.V. followed by 1.5 g every 4 h during labor or
- Clindamycin 900 mg I.V. every 8 h.

If chorioamnionitis is suspected broad spectrum antibiotic therapy including an agent active against GBS should replace GBS specific antibiotic prophylaxis.

Pediatrician should be present to clinically evaluate the baby after birth. Close supervision must be maintained for at least 12 h after delivery. If mother had ≥ 2 risk factors, blood cultures should be obtained and treatment started with Penicillin till culture results are available. Breastfeeding is not contraindicated.

3. **A 35-year-old primigravida has been referred to you because her routine anomaly scan at 20 weeks has shown presence of single choroid plexus cyst. Highlight the major issues involved in counseling.**

Choroid Plexus (CP) cysts are found in approximately 1% of routine second trimester scans.

The couple should preferably be counseled together and handled sympathetically. Specialist counseling should be adopted due to high levels of parental anxiety even after subsequent normal tests.

Choroids plexus cysts are considered 'Soft Markers' for fetal aneuploidy. These are usually transient ultrasound features which may indicate a risk of serious fetal chromosomal anomaly but which may in themselves be inconsequential.

Offer a detailed fetal anomaly scan to look for the presence of other soft markers (increased nuchal fold thickness, pyelectasis, hyperechogenic bowel, short femur, cardiac echogenic foci etc.) including the subtle ones like overlapping fingers, micrognathia, club foot and sandal gap. Dandy walker malformation should be specifically looked for. If expertise for the same does not exist in the current setup, she should be referred to a tertiary unit. Always offer a second opinion.

Presence of 2 or more markers increases the possibility of abnormal karyotype in fetus.

They usually resolve between 22-26 weeks gestation and are not usually associated with any other central nervous system problems or neurological sequelae.

Presence of isolated choroids plexus cysts increases an individual's prior risk of trisomy 18 by a factor of 9. Her risk of Down syndrome however remains the same.

Keeping her age in mind, offer Amniocentesis to determine fetal karyotype, since the age related risk for trisomy 18 is higher than the accepted threshold for amniocentesis (1 in 274). 1% fetal loss associated with amniocentesis should be explained to her and she should be allowed to make an informed decision.

Offer termination of pregnancy if abnormal karyotype is found. If she decides to continue the pregnancy, offer to arrange a meeting with a pediatrician.

Note: Any women >31 years with isolated CP cysts should be offered amniocentesis. If she is younger, and there are no other ultrasound features, karyotyping is not required as the accumulated risks due to amniocentesis are higher. Presence of single or multiple cysts or their subsequent disappearance do not alter the fetal prognosis. HCG values are lower on serum screening in trisomy 18.

4. **33-year-old primigravida presents at 16 weeks for her booking visit. She has a body weight of 140 kg and a body mass index of 40. She has no other apparent risk factor. What problems will you anticipate and counsel her for?**

Note: Divide the problems into antepartum, Intrapartum and Postpartum period. BMI values (weight in kg/height in m^2) are interpreted as follows:

< 15	Emaciation
15-20	Underweight
20-25	Desirable weight
25-30	Overweight
30 and above	Serious obesity.

Antepartum: Hypertensive disorders, diabetes, and urinary tract infection are common in obese women. Maternal blood pressure is difficult to determine when the upper arm is fat. Large cuffs should be used to prevent falsely high reading. Arrange for glucose tolerance test at booking and at 28 weeks. Screen for asymptomatic bacteriuria by culture and colony count of clean catch voided urine to screen for latent and overt urinary infections.

As the pregnancy proceeds it may be difficult to evaluate the size of fetus, presenting part, liquor estimation and fetal heart sounds by conventional means. Serial ultrasound scans may be required to evaluate fetal growth. Ultrasonic fetal weight assessments may be unreliable if too much adipose tissue in abdominal wall hampers visualization.

Dietary restrictions and excessive weight gain should be avoided. If required dietician's help should be sought. A daily exercise program should be adopted. There is no role of bypass or reductive surgeries in pregnancy.

During labor it may be mechanically difficult to site an intravenous cannula or an epidural catheter. Advance siting and involvement of senior obstetrician and anesthetist is desirable. Vigilance for Thrombophlebitis should be maintained.

Intrapartum monitoring may be difficult. Internal monitoring with fetal scalp electrodes is more appropriate. There may be Poor progress of labor because of persistently high head and occipito-posterior position due to excessive fat in ischiorectal fossa.

Postpartum hemorrhage, Low apgar scores, fetal macrosomia and shoulder dystocia are commonly associated. Good asepsis, prophylactic antibiotics and hemostasis should be maintained.

If cesarean section is required, both surgery and anesthesia is more hazardous. Regional analgesia should be preferred over general anesthesia. Delayed wound healing due to sweating, hematoma formation and diabetes is common. Single layer wound closure with nonabsorbable sutures is preferable. Placement of prophylactic surgical drains at wound site is debatable.

Deep vein thrombosis is more common in obese women. Early ambulation, TED stockings, and prophylactic heparin should be considered.

Neonate should be monitored for signs of hypoglycemia. Encourage early breastfeeding.

Adequate contraception before next pregnancy in the form of barriers, or intrauterine devices should be prescribed. Combined oral pills are a relative contraindication. She should be encouraged to loose weight before next pregnancy.

PAPER 3

1. Describe the use of Anti D.
2. Discuss management options for a primigravid women referred to your clinic with breech presentation at 38 weeks.
3. A routine anomaly scan performed at 18 weeks reveals an anterior abdominal defect in the fetus. How will you counsel the parents?
4. An epileptic woman controlled on carbamezipine and valproate wants to conceive and comes to you for advice. How will you counsel her? Briefly outline her antenatal and postnatal care.

1. Describe the use of Anti D.

Note: *Anti D use can be divided into prophylactic and therapeutic use. Further subdivision into usual and unusual dosage and route of administration can be planned. Use during Antenatal or postnatal period should be discussed. 99.2-99.3% women in UK have fetomaternal hemorrhage (FMH)< 4 ml at delivery. Upto 50% of larger FMHs occur after normal deliveries without any overt sensitizing event. Kleihauer acid elution test to detect fetal hemoglobin (Hb F), flow cytometry to detect RhD positive red cells or rosetting technique can be employed to detect FMH. Anticoagulated blood collected within 2 hrs of the event should be used.*

Anti D is prepared from immune plasma of human volunteers.

Anti D immunoglobulin (Ig) is given to **prevent** alloimmunisation resulting from feto maternal hemorrhages (FMHs) occurring in an RhD negative woman carrying an RhD positive fetus. Anti D is a blood product and women, especially JEHOVAH'S witness must make an informed decision prior to use.

Anti-D Ig should be given intramuscularly as soon as possible and within 72 h after the sensitizing event. If it is not given before 72 hours, a dose given within 9-10 days may provide some protection. Women who are already sensitized or have a weak expression of RhD (D^u) should not be given anti-D Ig.

Antenatally, at least 250 iu of Anti-D Ig should be given before 20 weeks' gestation and 500 IU thereafter. A test for the size of FMH is preferable when anti-D Ig is given after 20 weeks and additional doses given if required. It is used:

- Before 12 weeks if there has been uterine instrumentation. (Omit if no surgical intervention)
- Ectopic pregnancy
- Termination of pregnancy at any time (medical or surgical)
- Spontaneous complete or incomplete abortion after 12 weeks of pregnancy.
- Threatened miscarriage after 12 weeks. If bleeding continues intermittently, after 12 weeks, repeat anti D at 6 weekly interval.
- If uterine bleeding is very heavy and gestation is approaching 12 weeks, Anti D may be considered. Confirm period of gestation by ultrasound.
- Any time in pregnancy after the following potentially sensitizing events;
  - invasive prenatal diagnosis (amniocentesis, chorion villus sampling, fetal blood sampling)
  - other intrauterine procedures (e.g. insertion of shunts, embryo reduction)

- antepartum hemorrhage
- external cephalic version of the fetus
- closed abdominal injury
- intrauterine death
- Routine antenatal prophylaxis at 28 and 34 weeks with 500 IU decreases the incidence of alloimmunisation from 99.2 to 99.7%.

Postnatally: At least 500 IU of anti-D Ig must be given to every non-sensitized RhD negative woman within 72 hours following the delivery of an RhD positive infant. This includes women with alloantibodies other than anti-D. 500 IU of anti-D Ig is capable of suppressing immunization by 4-5 ml of RhD positive red cells. Test to detect FMH greater than 4 ml must also be undertaken, so that additional anti-D Ig can be given as appropriate.

If a woman has received inj anti D during pregnancy, she may have detectable anti D in her blood at delivery, anti-D Ig should be given to such women unless it has been clearly confirmed that she is already sensitized.

Therapeutic use: If an RhD negative woman requires platelet transfusion, RhD negative platelets should be transfused. If it is necessary to transfuse RhD positive platelets anti D prophylaxis with 250 IU should be given after every 3 adult doses of platelets as there may be some contamination from red cells (<0.1 ml RBC per vac).

Possible routes of administration: It is routinely administered as *Intramuscular injections*, best given into the deltoid muscle, (injections into the gluteal region often only reach the subcutaneous tissues and absorption may be delayed). Patients having marked thrombocytopenia should be given the anti-D Ig *subcutaneously* to avoid the possibility of a hematoma following intramuscular injection. *Intravenous* anti-D Ig is the preparation of choice when large volumes of Rh-positive blood has been transfused. The dose to be administered should assume that 500 IU of anti-D Ig IV will suppress immunization by 8-10 ml of fetal RBC. Intramuscular anti-D Ig must not be given intravenously. *Exchange transfusion* may be considered after adequate patient counseling when more than 2 units of RhD positive blood have been transfused.

2. Discuss management options for a primigravid women referred to your clinic with breech presentation at 38 weeks.

The prospective mother should be counseled regarding the presentation, various options for delivery and allowed to make an informed decision. Recent ultrasound (after 36 weeks) should be rechecked to confirm presentation, rule out placenta previa and fetal malformations. Adequacy of liquor, attitude of limbs (flexed, extended or footling) and head should be checked.

She should be offered **External Cephalic Version (ECV)** by appropriately trained professionals at 38 weeks. It should be performed on the labor ward, near to the facilities for emergency delivery. Ultrasound for guidance is helpful. Cardiotocography (CTG) before and after ECV reconfirms fetal well being. Tocolysis is effective both when used routinely or selectively. ECV carries a success rate of 40-60% and halves the rates of cesarean sections done for breech presentation.

Less than 1% will require emergency cesarean section for procedure related fetal distress, placental abruption and vaginal bleeding. Appropriate doses of injection Anti D (after Kleihauer count) should be administered to Rhesus negative women.

Postural management to promote cephalic version include knee chest position and elevation of pelvis using a cushion. It is popular but not very effective. **Moxibustion** is not a standard practice, but is known to be safe and may promote spontaneous version.

Elective cesarean section at 39 weeks is now considered the safest mode of delivery for a singleton, uncomplicated breech baby (Term breech trial). The chances of neonatal respiratory morbidity and mortality is decreased and there is a small chance of spontaneous correction of lie till that time. She still has around 70% chance of normal vaginal delivery in her next pregnancy.

The inherent risks of a surgical procedure, especially thromboembolism, bleeding and infection should be explained. If spontaneous labor starts before the scheduled surgery, emergency CS may be required which carries a higher morbidity.

Trial of vaginal delivery may be offered in the absence of any medical or obstetric complications. It carries higher risks of fetal morbidity and mortality and 20% women may still require emergency CS due to various reasons. Pelvimetry is not helpful in the prediction of cases suitable for vaginal delivery. If she still chooses to deliver vaginally or presents in advance labor, appropriately trained personnel should be present to conduct delivery.

Appropriate documentation of the counseling and women's decision should be made in her case records.

Note: 4% of all singleton pregnancies are breech presentations, the commonest reason being prematurity. Higher incidence of cerebral palsy in breech is related to prematurity and congenital malformations.

Moxibustion refers to burning of special herbs to stimulate the acupuncture points beside the outer corner of fifth toenail.

Contraindications to ECV include women in active labor, uterine scar or abnormality, fetal compromise, ruptured membranes, vaginal bleeding and medical conditions.

3. A routine anomaly scan performed at 18 weeks reveals an anterior abdominal defect in the fetus. How will you counsel the parents?

Parents should be dealt sympathetically and the differential diagnosis of such defects should be informed, i.e. gastroschisis, omphalocoele and hernia.

Omphalocele (exomphalos) is an hernia due to arrest of ventral medial migration of dermatomyotomes. 60-80% fetuses are associated with structural (esp. cardiac) or chromosomal anomalies. 1 in 6 babies will have abnormal karyotype, but for normal karyotypic fetuses survivability is around 75%.

Gastroschisis is a Paraumbilical defect of the anterior abdominal wall, usually considered a developmental accident. Less than 10% fetuses have associated anomalies, and only 1% have abnormal karyotype. The chances of a good outcome are very high with over 80% survival.

Further investigations, such as detailed ultrasound and fetal echo-cardiography should be arranged. Karyotyping should be offered.

Termination of pregnancy is an appropriate option before viability.

Parents should be offered extended counseling sessions with a multidisciplinary team comprising of an obstetrician with expertise in fetal medicine, a neonatal pediatrician, pediatric surgeon, clinical geneticist and anesthetist if they decide to continue pregnancy.

Information leaflets and illustrations showing pre- and postsurgery defects should be used at these sessions. Parents should be informed that baby may require prolonged hospital stay (up to 3 months) after birth and will require surgery to close the defect.

Serial ultrasound scans after 24 weeks to assess fetal growth, amniotic fluid volume and bowel appearance should be arranged.

Delivery should take place in a tertiary feto maternal unit with neonatal surgical facilities. Inducing preterm labor is not indicated and vaginal delivery is usually appropriate in the absence of medical or obstetric complications.

Risk of recurrence is usually less than 1%.

4. **An epileptic women controlled on carbamezapine and valproate wants to conceive and comes to you for advice. How will you counsel her? Briefly outline her antenatal and postnatal care.**

Conception should be delayed till epilepsy is well controlled and medical optimization have been achieved. If she has been seizure free for many years, reassure as majority (>50%) have a normal outcome. 25% women may experience an increased frequency of seizures in pregnancy.

There is no increased risk of miscarriage or obstetric complications due to epilepsy per se and there is no evidence of adverse effects of a single seizure on the fetus.

She should be advised to take 5 mg folic acid starting 3 months preconceptionaly till the end of pregnancy to counter the anti folate action of anticonvulsant drugs.

Neuro physician involvement should be sought to review necessity of anticonvulsant drugs and if possible to put her on monotherapy at lowest possible doses.

Risk of congenital malformations (GCA) should be discussed. Valproate (2%) and carbamezapine (1%) both can cause neural tube defects. Risk of GCA is higher (15%) with two drugs as compared to when she is controlled on single drug (6-7%). For valproate there is evidence of a dose dependent teratogenic effect. Risk of epilepsy in offspring should be explained and genetic counseling offered.

During her **antenatal** period risk of seizures, its implications for license and social security and the importance of compliance with medication and folic acid should be stressed. Prenatal diagnosis should be offered with maternal serum Alfa-feto-protein and detailed anomaly scan at 18-20 weeks. If required, monitor free drug levels; advise good diet, sleep and avoidance of precipitating factors. Offer multidisciplinary input with regular antenatal visits. Arrange regular growth scans if poorly controlled epileptic. Add oral Vitamin K 10 mg/day in the last 4 weeks to decrease the risk of hemorrhagic disease of newborn.

Postnatal: Neonate should also receive injection vit K. Encourage breast-feeding but monitor for signs of neonatal withdrawal or sedative effects. If dose of anticonvulsant was increased specifically during pregnancy, it should be reduced to pre- pregnancy doses gradually over 2-3 months. Avoid sleep deprivation and advice about avoidance of seizure related accidents.

Contraception with higher doses of oestrogens (50-100µgm) in combined pills is desirable. Efficacy of progesterone pill may be affected by hepatic enzyme inducers like carbamezapine. Barriers, Mirena (progesterone IUD) and progesterone injections are effective options. Valproate, clonazepam and newer drugs like vigabatrin, lamotrigine and gabapentin do not induce hepatic enzymes and all methods of contraception are suitable.

PAPER 4

1. Enumerate the predictors for shoulder dystocia and the manoeuver that you will attempt on encountering shoulder dystocia.

2. Enumerate the etiology, consequences of vaginal childbirth on pelvic floor and possible preventive strategies to minimize the damage.

3. Justify your management of confirmed spontaneous rupture of the membranes at 25 weeks gestation in a singleton pregnancy.

4. A primigravida at 13 weeks gestation presents at Accident and emergency with history of severe vomiting for the past one week. On examination she has tachycardia and dehydration. Discuss her management and possible complications.

1. **Enumerate the predictors for shoulder dystocia and the manoeuvers that you will attempt on encountering shoulder dystocia.**

It is difficult to predict shoulder dystocia. Majority occurs in infants less than 4.5 kg. Maternal diabetes, fetal macrosomia, previous history of shoulder dystocia (Recurrence risk 10%), prolonged labor, and delay in second stage are strong risk factors.

All the manoeuvers aim to increase the pelvic diameters and some reduce the biacromial diameter.

Call the senior obstetrician, SHO, midwife, neonatologist and anesthetist for help. Ask a junior midwife to note time of manoeuvers. Each manoevuer should be undertaken for 30 seconds.

Perform or extend episiotomy to create space for performing manoeuvers. Put your hand in the sacral hollow to find out the position of posterior shoulder.

With the help of two assistants, perform exaggerated flexion of maternal hips (McRobert's manoeuvre). This increases the anteroposterior diameter of maternal pelvis and may release the anterior shoulder without needing to do anything further.

Synchronize the maternal pushing with suprapubic pressure and gentle downward traction on the fetal head to force the anterior shoulder under the pubic symphysis.

Rotate the shoulders away from the anteroposterior diameter to facilitate delivery of posterior arm. Slide a hand in the sacral hollow behind the posterior shoulder and sweep the posterior arm across the fetal chest. Grasp the hand and deliver the posterior arm along with the head.

Attempt the Wood's corkscrew manoeuvre next by putting two fingers behind the posterior shoulder in an attempt to rotate it through 180 degrees. Since the pelvis is longer posteriorly, when the lower posterior shoulder reaches anteriorly, it becomes deliverable.

If the baby is still alive, cleidotomy or symphysiotomy can be tried by experienced operators. Zavanelli's manoeuvre to replace the head back into maternal abdomen and then delivering the baby by caesarean section has been successful in a few cases.

If there is no other option, manoeuvres can be repeated with the mother on all fours.

If the fetus dies during the manoeuvres, destructive procedures may be undertaken by an experienced operator.

Note: After the delivery of head, pH of the umbilical cord drops by 0.04/min. Interval between head and trunk delivery should be within 5 min.

2. Enumerate the etiology, consequences of vaginal childbirth on pelvic Floor and possible preventive strategies to minimize the damage.

The damage to perineum is maximum during the first delivery. Majority of vaginal deliveries are not followed by symptomatic damage to pelvic floor.

Perineal trauma at the time of vaginal delivery can cause increased incidence of dyspareunia, fistulae and perineal pain in the immediate postpartum period. Long-term pelvic sequelae can be urinary incontinence, anal incontinence and uterovaginal prolapse.

Vaginal delivery results in mechanical disruption of the pelvic floor and cause pudendal nerve injury resulting in urinary or anal incontinence or both. Women with inherent weakness of collagen within the pelvic floor may be at higher risk.

There are several aetiology mechanisms of pelvic floor injury.

A. Direct perineal trauma occurring from perineal laceration and episiotomy. Midline episiotomy has been associated with higher disruption of anal sphincter.

B. Muscle trauma secondary to maternal expulsive efforts and descent of fetal head causes a short-term decrease in pelvic floor strength.

C. Nerve damage due to compression effects may cause increased pudendal nerve latencies and denervation injury to pubococcygeus and external sphincter muscles.

D. Collagen and connective tissue changes during pregnancy and the repair of pelvic floor injury with weaker collagen leads to weakening of pelvic floor support mechanisms.

The **preventive strategies** include identification of "At risk women" in the antenatal period. This includes women who have experienced previous anal disruption, history of stress incontinence in self or mother prior to conception and collagen disorders.

Intrapartum: Preferential use of ventouse over forceps is less traumatic to perineum. Avoidance of difficult vaginal births and judicious use of elective caesarean section in selected cases (previous history of 3rd or 4th degree tears) is advocated. Restricted use of episiotomy, adequate training of doctors and midwives involved in repair of perineal trauma, and appropriate follow up of women with recognized anal sphincter trauma may help in decreasing the morbidity.

Postpartum: Standardized hospital protocols, treatment policies, good documentation and follow up should be available for women who develop postpartum incontinence and prolapse.

Education regarding reduction of family size, improved nutrition, pelvic floor exercises, avoidance of excessive weight gain and constipation to minimize the increase in intraabdominal pressure should be spread.

3. **Justify your management of confirmed spontaneous rupture of the membranes at 25 weeks gestation in a singleton pregnancy.**

Expectant management is the most favored for Premature rupture of membranes (PROM) between 24-31 weeks. The objective is to prolong pregnancy if there are no signs of fetal or maternal infection as the risks due to prematurity far outweigh the risks of subclinical infection. Nearly half of the babies born before 26 weeks gestation will have some form of disability (cerebral palsy, mental retardation) and, in 50% of these the disability will be severe **(EPICURE study)**.

Home management is increasingly seen as a safe protocol to adopt, particularly if there is no evidence of infection and onset of labor after one week of PROM and ultrasound shows adequate amniotic fluid volume. Parents should be counseled regarding fetomaternal monitoring and the likely mode of delivery, if expectant management is not considered appropriate.

Vigilance for chorioamnionitis should be maintained clinically (maternal fever, tachycardia, uterine pain/tenderness, purulent vaginal discharge) and by laboratory investigations (total and differential leukocyte count, C-reactive protein, amniotic fluid gram stain, microscopy and culture). High vaginal swab should be taken at presentation to look for bacterial vaginosis.

Serial tests for fetal well being; daily NST, twice weekly biophysical profile, weekly liquor volume and Doppler studies, fortnightly growth scans should be undertaken.

Avoid vaginal examinations to assess cervical status unless labor is established in order to prevent the increased risk of ascending infection.

An early aggressive broad spectrum intravenous antibiotic therapy is essential. It causes a significant reduction in perinatal mortality and morbidity, together with a reduction in maternal infectious morbidity and an improvement in latency to delivery.

A course of corticosteroids to induce fetal lung maturity is recommended in the absence of infection.

Tocolytics such as atosiban or nifedipine should be used until time is gained for corticosteroids to act or to facilitate fetomaternal transfer to tertiary center.

Continue pregnancy till signs of chorioamnionitis or fetal distress develop. Vaginal delivery is preferred except for breech presentation before 32 weeks. Cesarean section is reserved for usual obstetric indications. Outcome is improved if delivered in a center with good neonatal facilities. Pediatrician should be present at the time of delivery.

After delivery neonate should be screened for evidence of sepsis.

In the absence of a known etiology the recurrence risk is as high as 20-30%.

4. **A primigravida at 13 weeks gestation presents at A&E with history of severe vomiting for the past one week. On examination she has tachycardia and dehydration. Discuss her management and possible complications.**

Hyperemesis gravidarum is the likely diagnosis. History and clinical examination should be directed towards assessing her hydration status and ruling out other pathology like pyelonephritis, hepatitis, pancreatitis, diabetic ketoacidosis, thyrotoxicosis, gastroenteritis and drug induced vomiting.

She should be offered admission. Day care management is an accepted option for mild cases.

Investigations include; Full blood count for hematocrit and white cell count Blood urea and electrolytes, serum calcium, liver function and thyroid function tests (look for hyperthyroidism) in severe cases.

Urinalysis to exclude urinary tract infection, ketonuria.

Ultrasonography to exclude molar and multiple pregnancies.

On admission her weight, pulse and blood pressure should be recorded. Any emesis causing drugs should be suspended temporarily.

Keep her nil by mouth till vomiting is controlled. Multidisciplinary team may need to be involved in her care. Intravenous rehydration should be by normal saline or Hartmann's solution with added potassium chloride in each bottle. Thiamine 100 mg should be added weekly. Fluid and electrolyte regimens should be altered every day according to need. Attending staff should provide lots of encouragement, reassurance and psychological support.

Antiemetics; $5HT_3$ receptor antagonists (ondansetron) are effective in reducing nausea and vomiting. Pyridoxine is more effective in reducing severity of nausea. Ginger and P_6 acupressure are of proven benefit.

Antacids, H_2 receptor antagonists (Ranitidine) and Proton pump inhibitors (Omeprazole) may be added to prevent acid peptic disease.

Severe hyperemesis refractory to standard treatment may require total parentral nutrition, and corticosteroids. Upper GI endoscopy may be considered to rule out acid peptic disease, and oesophageal reflux. Termination of pregnancy can be offered in select cases.

Maternal complications that can complicate hyperemesis are oesophageal tears, hematemesis and Mallory-Weiss syndrome, Wernicke's encephalopathy, Korsakoff's psychosis, seizure and paralysis secondary to hyponatremia and hepatorenal failure.

Fetal complications are rare. Intrauterine growth restriction and fetal demise can happen in severe cases.

Note: The changes in blood chemistry with hyperemesis are as follows:

Hemoconcentration, leucocytosis, decrease in blood urea, hyponatremia, hypokalaemia, and hypochloraemic alkalosis, elevated liver enzymes and/or low TSH.

PAPER 5

1. Outline your management of a multiparous woman at 30 weeks gestation with a BP of 180/110 and ++ proteinuria. She has epigastric pain and right upper quadrant tenderness.
2. Summarize the options in managing a multiparous woman who has been found to have unstable lie at 38 weeks gestation.
3. Discuss the role of risk management in obstetrical practice.
4. Critically appraise the options of managing poor progress in the active phase of first stage in a primigravida who has spontaneous onset of labor at term.

1. **Outline your management of a multiparous woman at 30 weeks gestation with a BP of 180/110 and ++ protienuria. She has epigastric pain and right upper quadrant tenderness.**

This woman should be admitted in a high dependency unit close to labor ward. Obstetric registrar and consultant along with anesthesia registrar and senior labor room midwife should be informed about the case. Multidisciplinary treatment by involving surgeons (liver rupture), nephrologists (renal failure) and hematologists (coagulation defects) should be encouraged.

All maternal observations should be recorded meticulously. These include; blood pressure every 15 min, continuous pulse oxymetry, urine output (Foley's catheterization) and hourly temperature. Baseline blood investigations; full blood counts, serum urea, creatinine, electrolytes, liver function tests and urinalysis. Repeat them every 12-24 hrs as required. Peripheral blood smear to look for fragmented red blood cells, evidence of hemolysis and coagulation profile should be done. An electrocardiogram (EKG) should be recorded.

HELLP syndrome is the most likely diagnosis and delivery is the only definitive treatment. Ultrasound may need to be done to rule out other causes of upper abdominal pain.

Hypertension should be controlled by Hydralazine (5 mg i.v. rpt every 5 min, max 4 doses) or labetalol (20 mg i.v. rpt every 10 min in doubling dose till max 300 mg given). Add H_2 receptor antagonist (Ranitidine) to counter the side effects. If she settles down, labor ward protocol should be followed till delivery.

Fluid balance should be strictly monitored and maintained at 85 ml/hr. Prefer colloids. 500 ml human albumin solution (HAS) should be administered prior to hydralazine, cesarean section, if urinary output is <100 ml in 4 hrs and before regional anesthesia. CVP line should be inserted prior to giving HAS as risk of pulmonary oedema and fluid overload should be balanced with risk of acute renal failure due to hypovolemia.

If she gets a seizure, it should be controlled by magnesium sulphate. For every concurrent seizure 2 g bolus should be given iv. Serum magnesium levels should be considered if she has repeated seizures, absent deep tendon reflexes, spO_2 < 95% (Respiratory rate >14) and oliguria is present. Hospital protocols should be adhered to while deciding about use of prophylactic magnesium sulphate.

Fetal well being should be assessed be continuous electronic fetal monitoring, measuring amniotic fluid index, umbilical cord Doppler and growth scans if her condition allows.

Antenatal corticosteroids to enhance fetal lung maturity should be added but delivery should not be delayed for the sole purpose of buying time for steroids to act.

Coagulation defects should be corrected by infusions of Fresh Frozen plasma or platelet transfusions before delivery.

If maternal and fetal condition permits and Bishop Score is favorable, induction may be tried. If platelet count is $>100 \times 10^9$/l regional anesthesia is safe. Likelihood of cesarean section remains high and delivery should take place in a hospital with good neonatal facilities. Ergometrine should be avoided in the post partum period and intensive monitoring should continue for 72 hrs.

Risk of recurrence is high-up to 40%.

2. Summarize the options in managing a multiparous woman who has been found to have unstable lie at 38 weeks gestation.

History should be checked to confirm dates, relevant past obstetric (previous modes of delivery), family history and gestational diabetes ruled out.

A rough estimate of amniotic fluid should be made clinically. A pelvic examination should be done in the absence of placenta previa to identify any obstruction in pelvis (Tumor or fibroid) and to assess the Bishop's score.

Ultrasound should be done to measure amniotic fluid index (AFI), placental localization and fetal well being.

Woman should be counseled about the options available; expectant and active management and she should be allowed to make an informed decision.

Expectant Mx: In 8 out of 10 cases the lie becomes longitudinal without any intervention at the onset of labor. There is a risk of cord prolapse in cases of spontaneous rupture of membranes and at onset of labor and the need for prompt hospitalization should be made clear. Maintaining knee – chest position for a few hours every day has been advocated by some but not fully tested.

Active management involves hospitalization from 37 weeks onwards. Daily observations for feto-maternal well being and prompt diagnosis of labor or rupture of membranes are made. Once longitudinal lie is established and maintained for 48 hrs she may be discharged home to await spontaneous labor.

Woman can be offered ultrasound guided external cephalic version (ECV) once she is admitted. If longitudinal lie is established and maintained she may be discharged. Anti D prophylaxis and fetal monitoring should be used accordingly. Alternatively, after ECV a stabilizing induction with titrated intravenous oxytocin drip is started followed by amniotomy once active labor is established.

She should be given the option of elective cesarean section performed at 38-39 weeks, ideally after converting the lie to longitudinal, or if ECV fails or due to associated medical of obstetrical factors.

When the membranes rupture or labor begins and the lie is longitudinal, labor should be managed as per normal after exclusion of cord presentation/ prolapse. If the lie is not longitudinal, emergency cesarean section or external version are two options. There is no role of internal podalic version in singleton pregnancies.

3. Discuss the role of risk management in obstetrical practice.

Risk management involves methods for early identification of adverse events, using either staff reports or systematic screening of records followed by creation of a database to identify common patterns and develop a system of accountability to prevent future incidents (RCOG).

The common aim is to reduce harm to patients, relatives and staff at workplace. When mishaps occur, the potential for damage is minimized.

Good hospital risk management has been found to decrease the frequency of adverse events, reduces the chance of a medicolegal claim being made and controls the cost of claims that are being made. It incorporates a no blame culture and focuses on developing a system of accountability to prevent future incidents. It is an approach to enhancing the overall quality of care with special emphasis on care episodes with unexpected outcomes.

Risk identification can be by reporting all adverse trigger events by means of incident forms, which should then be reviewed by experts in a risk management committee **(Risk analysis)**. Computerization of maternity information system greatly enhances the efficiency of incident reporting.

In UK a recent website has been launched for anonymous reporting of incidents called NPSA (National Patient safety agency).

Hospital policies, protocols and guidelines should be maintained and regularly updated *(Risk control)*. All new incumbents should be introduced to them. Structured proformas should be available for standard clinical situations. There should be regular teaching (CTG learning sessions, CME), training (instrumental delivery, cesarean section skills), drills and skills sessions (shoulder dystocia) for the junior staff and midwives. Adequate staffing (40 hr labor ward consultant cover, 1.15 midwives per woman in labor, and junior staffing) should be encouraged. Professional assessment of all staff should be maintained periodically. Regular clinical audits to assess existing standards should be undertaken.

Labor room should have an identified lead midwife and obstetrician who would be responsible for its smooth functioning. They should encourage good documentation with properly signed and dated entries in labor record.

Good communication between woman, her partner and health professionals at all levels is essential.

An efficient complaints procedure should exist in all hospitals and accessible to women who want to complaint. Staff should be encouraged to de-brief women about their management.

Clear hospital policies regarding *funding* for litigation claims and insurance should exist.

4. Critically appraise the options of managing poor progress in the active phase of first stage in a primigravida who has spontaneous onset of labor at term.

When the rate of cervical dilatation is less than 1 cm/hr in the active phase, poor progress should be diagnosed. Partograms used to monitor labor can help to select cases requiring intervention and augmentation of labor.

Inefficient uterine contractions are recognized as the commonest cause for poor progress. Cephalopelvic disproportion, malposition (most likely occipito transverse or occipito posterior position) and malpresentation must be ruled out by accurate assessment prior to any intervention. Urine should be checked for ketones.

Conservative management with adequate hydration, nutrition, analgesia, reassurance and watchful expectancy is appropriate if maternal and fetal condition is satisfactory. Presence of a supportive companion and ambulation during labor has been shown to result in shorter labors.

Approximately half of the women deemed to have slow progress perform equally well regardless of management strategy.

Active management comprises of amniotomy, early use of oxytocin, and continuous professional support to ensure optimal progress of labor and normal delivery. It decreases the risk of prolonged labor and associated morbidity of maternal infection, uterine rupture, post partum hemorrhage and maternal death. The total duration of labor may be shortened by 60-120 min.

Active management is ineffective in reducing the rate of Cesarean section or operative vaginal delivery. Early amniotomy leads to reduction in the duration of labor by 60-90 min, but may increase the risk of infection.

Injudicious use of oxytocin may cause intrapartum fetal hypoxia and maternal hyponatremia. Continuous fetal monitoring with CTG is neccessary and good analgesia is advisable with oxytocin infusions. Optimal interval between dose increments is 30 min and dose should be started at 10 miu/ml and titrated to achieve a contraction frequency of 4 in 10 min each lasting >40 s.

Allow the woman to make an informed decision after full discussion of the management options. Some women resent any interventions. Reassessment by vaginal and abdominal examinations must be done at appropriate intervals according to the hospital protocols, to establish the success of adopted option.

If despite adequate trial of oxytocin, there is no progress, cesarean section should be performed.

PAPER 6

1. Debate the use of routine early pregnancy ultrasound.
2. An anxious 14 weeks pregnant school teacher presents at your outpatient clinic. One child in her class has been diagnosed to be suffering from Varicella. Discuss the advice you will give her.
3. A 24-year-old parous woman complaint of painful intercourse 6 weeks after childbirth. How will you manage her?
4. A 20-year-old multigravida repeatedly presents at A&E with concerns about loss of fetal movements. All the preliminary tests of fetal well being are unremarkable. While you were reassuring her, she reveals that her husband is an alcoholic and abuses her. Briefly outline your management plan.

1. **Debate the use of routine early pregnancy ultrasound.**

Note: The essay plan for all debate questions should be divided into pros and cons of subject matter.

Pros: Early pregnancy scan provides with good dating to establish period of gestation accurately. This is especially useful if date of last menstrual cycle is not known accurately or she has poor dates due to irregular cycles, use of pills, and conception in immediate post partum period. Dating by LMP (Naegele method) is inaccurate in 20% women. Timing and interpretation of test results of serum screening depends on accurate knowledge of gestational age. Accurate dating has been shown to decrease rate of labor inductions (up to 40%) and cesarean sections for post dated pregnancies. Timing of induction of labor or elective CS depends critically on accurate timing.

Early confirmation of fetal location and viability is reassuring to many women at high-risk (previous ectopic, recurrent early miscarriages).

Determination of chorionicity in multiple pregnancies is easier and accurate in first trimester. Early detection of higher order multiple pregnancies provides opportunities for fetal reduction.

Nuchal translucency measurement at 11-14 weeks has been recommended by the RCOG as part of screening program for detection of Down's syndrome.

Early detection of gross unsuspected fetal malformations may permit early surgical termination of pregnancy and decreased associated morbidity. Majority of central nervous system defects, neck anomalies, gastrointestinal and renal defects can be detected in a first trimester scan. Majority of first trimester terminations are done by suction evacuation, hence making the pathological confirmation of anomaly more difficult and time consuming.

Cons: The earlier in the first trimester the scan is performed, the greater are the chances of picking up pathological pregnancies which would have failed otherwise also. Hence, it may be argued as a futile exercise and financial drain.

Routine scanning of all pregnant women will increase requirement of trained manpower in the institutions. The cost effectiveness of routine screening needs to be assessed at hospital level.

Most women in under resourced/developing countries may not book early enough for antenatal care and hence miss an opportunity for the scan.

All congenital malformations are not detected by a first trimester scan. Spina bifida, heart and limb malformations may require a second trimester scan.

There is no consensus on when to perform the early scan. Dating is more accurate when established at 8-10 weeks. Details of fetal anatomy are better visualized at 13 weeks.

2. **An anxious 14 weeks pregnant school teacher presents at your outpatient clinic. One child in her class has been diagnosed to be suffering from Varicella. Discuss the advice you will give her.**

Note: The essay plan can be divided into immediate advice, advice for later on in pregnancy and advice upon delivery.

The incubation period of chicken pox is 14-21 days and the period of infectivity is from 48 hours prior to eruption of rash till vesicles crust over in average 6 days. It is a DNA virus of herpes family and spreads due to droplet infection, fomites, direct contact with vesicular fluid and transplacental transmission.

Immediate advice: Details of contact history, degree of exposure and past history of varicella in the woman should be enquired. Most women (90%) are already IgG seropositive and hence immune. Primary varicella infection is rare in pregnancy especially in women with children and if history of previous exposure is present, she should be reassured.

With no previous history of exposure or doubtful immune status, varicella Zoster IgG titers should be checked. This should preferably be arranged from serum saved at booking. She should avoid contact with other pregnant women and immunocompromised population till the result is known. If the consultation is at GP level, she should not be sent to maternity hospital for investigations.

If the patient is not immune and develops primary varicella Zoster infection or shows serological evidence of seroconversion, she should be informed about a 2% risk of congenital varicella syndrome (FVS) in the fetus. There is no increase in spontaneous miscarriage rate.

Advice during pregnancy: A detailed ultrasound should be arranged at 18-20 weeks (or after 5 weeks of exposure) to detect changes in the fetus. FVS consists of skin scarring, eye defects (micropthalmia, chorioretinitis, cataracts), limb hypoplasia, and neurological abnormalities (microcephaly, cortical atrophy, optic atrophy, bladder and bowel sphincter dysfunction).

Fetal blood sampling to demonstrate Varicella IgM in suspicious fetuses can be offered if parents are very anxious and are willing to accept the risks of cordocentesis and termination.

One in ten affected women may develop pneumonia, hepatitis or encephalitis with a severe infection or if she is immunocompromised. Oral acyclovir is safe in pregnancy and decreases the severity of infection. If she presents within 10 days of exposure, and is not immune, she should be given Zoster immune globulin 0.2-0.4 mg/kg.

Advice upon delivery: Neonate should be examined by ophthalmologist after birth.

3. A 24-year-old parous woman complaint of painful intercourse 6 weeks after childbirth. How will you manage her?

Management should focus on the underlying cause. **Establish if it is a pre-existing cause, related to delivery trauma, or due to breast-feeding dryness.** Other Secondary causes include physical problems like pelvic adhesions, PID, cervicitis, cystitis, scar tissue, and severe constipation etc; Psychological trauma, and decreased libido.

Her own perspective of her problem, order of its development, social and family demands, privacy, financial support and availability of help at home, fear of pain and pregnancy, previous history of depression should be elicited. **History** of any hormonal contraceptives being used, type and details of delivery, her experience during childbirth, breastfeeding and details of pain (on entry or deep) should be asked in a sensitive and non judgmental manner.

She should be reassured about decreased sexual interest after childbirth as >50% women report loss of sexual desire and discomfort on resuming sexual activity. Prompt and adequate management of pain is essential to prevent long-term physical and psychosocial morbidity.

Inspect the lower genital tract for any swelling, irritation, warts, varicosities, abrasions, poor anatomical alignment of perineal tears or episiotomy and scar tissue bands. Assisted vaginal delivery is more likely to be associated with perineal trauma.

Gentle per speculum examination and **swabs** should be taken if infection is suspected. **Examination** should first include single finger insertion to rule out vaginismus and to avoid confusion with pelvic pain. Bimanual examination to elicit cervical excitation, and evidence of pelvic infection should be done with good lubrication.

Pelvic **ultrasound** should be asked for if any pelvic pathology is suspected.

Provide Reassurance if due to tiredness or increased demands on her time. Water based lubricant jelly should be prescribed to relieve vaginal dryness associated with breastfeeding. Modified Fenton's procedure and perineal refashioning should be offered for excessive scar tissue.

Changing the positions of intercourse may be advisable for deep dyspareunia. Adequate contraception should be prescribed. If preexisting or non organic cause is found she should be referred to psychosexual therapist.

Refractory cases may be referred to dedicated perineal care clinics with multidisciplinary input.

4. **A 20-year-old multigravida repeatedly presents at A&E with concerns about loss of fetal movements. She is currently 30 weeks in gestation. All the preliminary tests of fetal well being are unremarkable. While you were reassuring her, she reveals that her husband is an alcoholic and abuses her. Briefly outline your management plan.**

She should be handled sympathetically and calmly, with a non judgmental approach.

Total confidentiality of the conversation should be assured. It is important to convey that she is being understood and taken seriously.

Details about her family background, educational status, social and financial support should be enquired to give her practical suggestions. High risk behavior should be identified by personal history of alcoholism, drug abuse, multiple sexual partners, treatment for depression and unwanted pregnancy. Any perceived threats to her or her children's life should be directly asked.

Reassure her that it is not her fault that she is being abused and she must not allow the situation to continue. Domestic violence is on the increase and appropriate support is available.

She should be encouraged to talk to someone in the family or friend whom she trusts.

She can contact the domestic violence unit of local police for protection. Local women's aid groups can provide assistance with employment and temporary shelters. All possible help to get contact numbers should be provided. The police can be informed from the hospital on her behalf. In emergency situations short term hospital admission may be offered. She can prepare an escape plan with her children.

Her complaints should be documented with her prior consent. General practitioner and area social worker should be involved.

Follow up appointment should be arranged in the outpatient setting to reassure her about fetal well being. Vigilance should be observed for obstetric complications like prematurity and abruption.

PAPER 7

1. A primigravida has been referred to you at 41 weeks by the GP. Discuss the management options.
2. A primigravida with 32 weeks pregnancy presents at A&E with high grade fever, headache and malaise. She is pale, icteric and has enlarged liver and spleen. Other systemic examination is unremarkable. She has just returned from a family vacation in Africa. Discuss the relevant management issues.
3. You are asked to see a 16-year-old girl in the early weeks of pregnancy. How will her young age alter your subsequent care?
4. A 33-year-old woman noticed a small breast lump on her left breast one weak back. She is currently 16 weeks pregnant and is very concerned as her maternal aunt had died of breast cancer. How will you manage her condition?

1. **A primigravida has been referred to you at 41 completed weeks by the GP. Discuss the management options.**

The management options are active induction of labor after 41 weeks or expectant management with regular fetal monitoring.

Establish accurate dates from her previous records, ideally from first trimester ultrasound. Dating by LMP alone has a tendency to overestimate gestational age. She should be reevaluated for any fetal or maternal risk factors necessitating urgent intervention.

Women with uncomplicated pregnancies should be counseled for relative risks and benefits of induction vs. expectant management. Her wishes, cervical scoring and availability of ante partum testing facilities should be taken into consideration when management is planned.

Beyond 41 weeks, the incidence of meconium staining of amniotic fluid, need for intrapartum fetal blood sampling, shoulder dystocia, fetal hypoxia and fetal death increase due to uteroplacental insufficiency. There are increased rates of neonatal seizure and death. Delivery at 42 weeks was associated with doubling of perinatal mortality rate compared with delivery at 39-41 weeks.

There are increased risks of instrumental and operative delivery and hemorrhage in the mother with an overall increase in maternal mortality. Maternal anxiety increases as she passes her estimated date of delivery.

In an uncomplicated pregnancy, she should be offered induction of labor beyond 41 weeks. Prior to formal induction of labor, woman should be offered a vaginal examination for membrane sweep. Nipple stimulation is an alternative if examination is refused.

From 42 weeks, women who decline induction of labor should be offered increased antenatal monitoring consisting of at least twice weekly Cardiotocography and ultrasound estimations of maximum amniotic fluid pool depth. She should be informed that monitoring may not be effective in reducing the incidence of 'postmature' fetal deaths.

Labor can be induced with prostaglandin E_2 pessaries (3 mg), followed if necessary by oxytocin and artificial rupture of membranes.

Labor should be monitored by continuous fetal heart rate monitoring and reviewed frequently. Amnioinfusion may be considered for meconium staining of liquor or FHR abnormalities associated with oligohydramnios.

In the presence of coexisting medical or obstetrical complicating factors cesarean section should be performed.

Note: Term traditionally means period of gestation from 37 weeks plus 6 days till 40 weeks +7 days (37 completed weeks to 41 weeks).

2. **A primigravida with 32 weeks pregnancy presents at A&E with high grade fever, headache and malaise. She is pale, icteric and has enlarged liver and spleen. Other systemic examination is unremarkable. She has just returned from a family vacation in Africa. Discuss the relevant management issues.**

History: There should be a high index of suspicion for Malaria on account of her travel history. The predominant symptoms are fever, rigors, nausea, abdominal pain, bodyache and headache. Look for Pallor, Jaundice, moderate and tender hepatosplenomegaly on **examination**.

Investigations: Diagnosis is made by detection of parasites on peripheral blood smear. Thick smear is required for diagnosis and thin film for identification of species. Samples should be withdrawn 4-6 hours after spike of temperature due to increased parasitemia at that time. Serial samples may be required for diagnosis. Parasites in >2% red cells indicate severe infection. A simple and rapid Dipstick immunological test is reserved for P. falciparum infection. Full blood counts, hematocrit, platelet count, renal functions, liver enzymes and blood sugar should be checked periodically. HIV testing should be offered.

Maternal **complications** include; hypoglycemia, severe anemia, pulmonary edema, acute renal failure, hepatitis, hyperpyrexia, cerebral malaria, hemorrhagic and septicemic shock.

There are higher chances of intrauterine fetal hyperpyrexia causing preterm labor, fetal acidosis and still births. 1% babies are born with congenital malaria and may have fever, irritability, feeding problems, anemia, and jaundice and hepatosplenomegaly.

Supportive management involves appropriate airway protection, fluid replacement while watching for development of pulmonary edema and hypoglycemia.

Fever should be tackled by adequate exposure, fans, tepid sponging, and paracetamol.

Blood transfusion for severe anemia and dialysis for renal failure should be available.

Cerebral malaria is a medical emergency with 15-20% mortality rates. Intensive care treatment and multidisciplinary approach is essential. I.V. antibiotics along with antimalarials should be given due to increased susceptibility of pneumococcal and gram negative septicemia.

Fetal surveillance with antenatal corticosteroids, daily nonstress test and serial ultrasounds should be maintained. Cord blood smear should be taken after delivery to rule out congenital malaria.

Treatment should be by most effective antimalarial drug available. Choice of drug depends on pattern of local drug resistance, disease severity, drug safety and availability. Falciparum malaria may be multi drug resistant.

Chloroquine is the drug of choice for *P. vivax, P. malariae and P. ovale.* Quinine is more effective against *P. falciparum.* Both are safe for use in pregnancy. Mefloquine, Pyrimethamine with sulfadoxine and Artemisinins are second line drugs.

Primaquine is contraindicated in pregnancy but is safe during breastfeeding. Safety of newer drugs i.e. halofentrine, lumefantrine; atovaqunone has not been established in pregnancy.

Indications for urgent delivery are mainly acute fetal distress. Pediatrician should be present at the time of delivery and congenital malaria ruled out.

Note: *Malaria spreads by bite of female anopheles mosquitoes, rarely by blood transfusion, vertical transmission and needle stick injury.*

Paroxysms of fever are typical of the species;

Every 48 hours – *P. vivax* and *P. ovale.*

36-48 hours – *P. falciparum.*

72 hours – *P. malariae.*

80% of global malaria burden occurs in Sub Saharan Africa.

3. **You are asked to see a 15-year-old girl in the early weeks of pregnancy. How will her young age alter your subsequent care?**

Majority of teenage pregnancies may be unwanted and unplanned. They usually have poor compliance with antenatal care and should be encouraged for regular attendance.

Healthy eating habits should be stressed to avoid risk of nutritional deficiencies. Adequate supplements should be prescribed.

Early pregnancy ultrasound scan should be done to confirm gestational age.

Associated cigarette smoking, alcohol consumption and recreational drug use are common amongst pregnant adolescents. A specific risk and need analysis should be done early and interventional strategies sought.

Risk of sexually transmitted diseases is higher as she may not be in a stable relationship. If positive, referral to genitourinary clinics and appropriate contact tracing should be advised. Tests for Chlamydia, HIV, and syphilis should be offered.

Antepartum: Medical complications include anemia, urinary tract infection, hypertension, and preterm labor. She should be handled sympathetically and enquiries should be made about perceived social isolation and financial difficulties. Multidisciplinary team with a social worker, family doctor and a dedicated midwife should be involved in her care. Special care should be given to allow her to continue her education at school or by a home tutor.

Information leaflets about pregnancy, breastfeeding, delivery and child rearing should be provided. She should be encouraged to involve and confide in family members or friends whom she trusts.

Intrapartum: They have higher analgesia requirement and operative assistance during labor. Shoulder dystocia and obstructed labor is a possibility, keeping the small pelvis in mind. Involvement of partner or family members for psychological support during labor should be promoted. If her physical development is still immature, she should be referred to an equipped unit for delivery.

Postpartum: There is a shorter interval to next pregnancy, low birth weight babies and sudden infant death syndrome. After delivery, feeding practices, infant safety, (child protection issues, possible abuse) social and financial concerns should be discussed openly. Effective contraception should be advised and adequate supplies issued if required. Use of condoms should be encouraged to prevent sexually transmitted diseases.

4. **A 33-year-old woman noticed a small breast lump on her left breast one week back. She is currently 16 weeks pregnant and is very concerned as her maternal aunt had died of breast cancer. What is your initial management of her problem?**

The majority (90%) of breast lumps have benign pathology. Triple assessment by clinical examination, imaging and cytology is the basis for diagnosis of any breast lesion.

History about associated features like pain, nipple discharge, and previous breast disease, use of pills and details of family history should be enquired.

Examination of both breasts should include inspection, and palpation of lump to estimate its size, position, consistency, fixity and any overlying skin changes. Axillary and supraclavicular lymph nodes should be palpated for enlargement. Physiological changes in the breast during pregnancy make clinical examination more difficult and inaccurate.

Investigations: Ultrasound of breast is useful to differentiate cystic and solid masses. Mammography under 35 year should be used only when clearly indicated. It can be safely performed during pregnancy but it has limited use due to hyperemia and edema in breast tissue.

Fine needle aspiration cytology or biopsy should be performed whenever indicated for accurate cytological diagnosis. Woman should be informed about the risk of bleeding, infection and milk fistulas.

If it is a benign lump, she should be reassured as such and advised for follow up after delivery.

If malignancy is detected, a complete physical examination, blood testing and chest radiograph should be performed. MRI to detect metastasis is safe for both mother and fetus. Multidisciplinary treatment with obstetrician, breast surgeons and clinical oncologist should be incorporated.

There is no evidence that termination of pregnancy after detection of breast carcinoma is necessary to improve prognosis. However treatment during pregnancy will require clear discussions between the woman and her care giver team on the relative benefits of early delivery followed by treatment vs. commencement of therapy while continuing the pregnancy. Termination of Pregnancy should be offered if the woman so wishes. 5 year survival in node negative women is close to 90% but two thirds of women have advanced disease at the time of detection.

Surgery is usually the first line **treatment** with mastectomy or lumpectomy and axillary clearance being the first option deferring reconstruction. Combination chemotherapy with 5-Fluorouracil, doxorubicin, and cyclophosphamide given for 4-6 cycles is safe after the first trimester.

Radiotherapy should be preferably deferred in pregnancy. If absolutely essential, appropriate thickness of lead shield to decrease fetal doses should be used. Serum CA153 is used for follow up in pregnancy.

Long-term survival after breast cancer does not seem to be affected by pregnancy. She can safely breast feed from the unaffected breast if not on any toxic drugs.

PAPER 8

1. A 28-year-old woman who had an epidural for analgesia in labor was delivered with forceps. After removal of her urinary catheter she is unable to void. Discuss her subsequent management.
2. There has been an outbreak of B-19 parvovirus infection in a nursery school and a school teacher at 13 weeks gestation is worried about the implications on her pregnancy. Discuss the issues involved.
3. A 32-year-old multigravida woman has had a clot in her leg two years back. She is currently 8 weeks pregnant. How will this information change your management of the remainder of her pregnancy?
4. A 37-year-old woman conceives following infertility treatment. A scan at 10 weeks shows quadruplets. How would you counsel her?

1. **A 28-year-old woman who had an epidural for analgesia in labor was delivered with forceps. After removal of her urinary catheter she is unable to void. Discuss her subsequent management.**

Management includes finding out the reason for her problem (structural/neurological/infective/pre-existing/pregnancy related) and then administrating specific treatment. General measures should be adopted till then to provide relief to the patient.

Operative delivery, prolonged labor and epidural analgesia all predispose to postpartum urinary retention which can be associated with long term bladder dysfunction.

History: Review labor records and time of last epidural top up. Prolonged labor can cause devascularization and laceration bladder neck injury with outflow obstruction. Rule out any past urinary dysfunction.

Examine her hydration status to rule out hypovolemia and palpate bladder intra abdominally. Examine the perineum for any periurethral tears, painful episiotomy, and vulval hematoma. Check for urethral integrity, the sphincter may be damaged during repair of a tear in proximity or involved in a laceration.

Treatment: Pass a Foley's catheter, and if the drained urine volume is more than 400 cc, continuous bladder drainage should be provided and kept in situ for at least 12 hours.

Fluid balance chart should be maintained for least 24 hours after delivery in all cases of operative delivery. A catheter sample should be checked for urine infection. Multidisciplinary input may be required by involving a urologist and anesthetist. Carbachol may be of benefit in select cases.

Provide reassurance and adequate analgesia.

Prolonged urinary retention may require urodynamic investigations and intermittent self catheterization or suprapubic catheterization. She should be offered physiotherapy-directed strategies to prevent urinary incontinence.

2. **There has been an outbreak of B-19 parvovirus infection in a nursery school and a school teacher at 13 weeks gestation is worried about the implications on her pregnancy. Discuss the issues involved.**

In school outbreaks one thirds of susceptible staff contracts B 19 infection. Vertical transmission occurs in 30% of these maternal infections and may result in severe fetal infections. Being in constant touch with small children at workplace or home increases her susceptibility to acquire B19 infection.

25% of all infections in adults are asymptomatic. Fever, malaise, arthralgia, and hemolytic anemia may be the presenting symptoms in adults and should be treated symptomatically.

Infected fetuses may develop chronic hemolytic anemia, non immune hydrops fetalis, myocarditis, intrauterine fetal death or still birth. Hydrops due to B19 infection has a good prognosis and resolves spontaneously in one third cases.

Determine her serostatus for B19 parvovirus. In the presence of IgG and absence of IgM, she should be reassured as she is **immune to infection**. If she is **susceptible** (IgG negative, IgM negative), but not yet infected, consideration may be given to exclude her from classrooms till she is 20 weeks of gestation. Repeat testing 3 weeks later.

If maternal **infection is confirmed** (IgM positive), serial ultrasound scans should be done to detect fetal hydrops at the earliest. Referral to a tertiary fetal medicine unit should be done once fetal hydrops is diagnosed. Infection in pregnancy is not an indication for therapeutic termination.

Fetal blood sample should be taken to assess the degree of anemia. If severe, intrauterine blood transfusions and early delivery after a course of steroids is advised. Conservative management and reassessment is appropriate if anemia is mild and fetal reticulocyte count is high.

Note: *Parvovirus B 19 has single stranded DNA and causes 'slapped cheek'/ fifth disease (erythema infectiosum) in childhood. Periods of increased activity are seen during late summer and early spring, every 3-4 years in UK. Transmission is through respiratory secretions, parenteral and vertical routes. Incubation period is 5-10 days. Rash occurs 1-5 days after disappearance of viremia and person is non infective at the time of symptoms.*

IgG usually persists for life after acquiring infection and conveys lasting immunity to further infection. ELISA, RIA, PCR can be used to detect viral DNA.

3. **A 32-year-old multigravida woman has had a clot in her leg two years back. She is currently 8 weeks pregnant. How will this information change your management of the remainder of her pregnancy?**

Details of her previous illness, treatment taken and duration of treatment should be enquired. Detailed medical records for the diagnosis should be asked for and the concerned physician should be contacted if possible. The diagnosis of past venous thromboembolism should be assumed if good history of prolonged anticoagulation is available.

A need and risk assessment should be done at the earliest by detailed history and risk factors for thromboembolism. The assessment should be repeated as the pregnancy advances.

She has an increased incidence of recurrence in present pregnancy and the risk is proportional to the reason for previous VTE.

She should be offered screening for inherited and acquired thrombophilia if not tested before. Multidisciplinary approach with hematologist should be adopted.

If previous VTE was associated with pregnancy, more than one episode of VTE, positive family history, an identifiable thrombophilia or recurrent risk factor (obesity), she should be offered antenatal prophylaxis with heparin. The prophylaxis should start as early as possible and continue throughout pregnancy. Low dose aspirin should be added in women with Antiphospholipid syndrome. Warfarin is contraindicated in the first trimester due to risk of teratogenesis and should preferably be avoided in pregnancy.

Immobilization during pregnancy, labor and the puerperium should be minimized and dehydration should be avoided. She should be encouraged to wear Graduated elastic compression stockings (TED) throughout their pregnancy and for 6-12 weeks after delivery.

At the onset of labor she should be advised, not to inject any further heparin. She should be reassessed by senior anesthetist, hematologist and obstetrician regarding further dose and timing of heparin.

If she has received regional analgesia, LMWH should be withheld until 4 hours after insertion or removal of epidural catheter.

Women with previous VTE and no thrombophilia should be offered prophylaxis with low molecular weight heparin (LMWH) for 6 weeks after delivery. In women with identifiable thrombophilia, the duration of postnatal prophylaxis depends on specific thrombophilia and varies from 6-12 weeks. In women with high risk of coagulopathy (APH, PPH, wound hematoma), unfractionated heparin should be used for thromboprophylaxis.

Combined oral contraceptives should be avoided. Breastfeeding is safe with LMWH and warfarin.

Note: *The risk factors for thromboembolism include pregnancy, previous VTE, congenital and acquired thrombophilia, obesity, high parity, medical and pregnancy related diseases causing increased viscosity of blood. Pulmonary thromboembolism is the commonest direct cause of maternal death in UK. Risk is highest in the immediate puerperium, following vaginal delivery, with obesity and age >35 years being the common risk factors.*

Side effects of heparin include—Bleeding from overdose, thrombocytopenia, osteoporosis, alopecia (transient and reversible) hypersensitivity reactions. All are less with LMWH. It does not cross the blood brain barrier and placenta. There is a 2% risk of wound hematoma on heparin.

4. A 37-year-old woman conceives following infertility treatment. A scan at 10 weeks shows quadruplets. How would you counsel her?

Careful history including ease of conception, parity, and nature of treatment for infertility should be enquired. Both the partners should preferably be present at the time of counseling.

The options include non intervention, selective termination or termination of pregnancy. Couple's moral and religious stance on the subject should be taken into consideration.

With **non intervention**, there is a high chance of loss of all fetuses which may be unacceptable to women with long history of primary infertility, especially as further conception may progressively become difficult. Possibility of prolonged hospital stay, higher incidence of preterm births and its sequelae like cerebral palsy should be discussed. Huge financial and psychological impact of multiple births on the family unit may be unacceptable. Referral to equipped center with facilities for neonatal intensive care may be required.

Termination of pregnancy may be acceptable in women with secondary infertility, to minimize the impact on the rest of the family.

Multifetal pregnancy reduction (MFPR) may be offered between 10-13 weeks. Instillation of 0.5-1.5 ml of Potassium chloride within fetal thorax by trans abdominal approach remains the most favored option. Nuchal translucency should be measured in all embryos. Embryos having significant risk of aneuploidies or monoamniotic twins are selected for reduction. In the absence of detectable anomalies, choice is based on ease of approach. Embryos close to cervix are avoided. The technical success rate is close to 100%.

There is a chance of spontaneous loss of an embryo adding to the risk of losing the remaining embryos. After 13 weeks, the chance of spontaneous loss is small. A small theoretical risk of infectious necrosis and DIC remain. Procedure related pregnancy loss rates vary with no. of fetuses reduced and is 5-10%. There is a higher chance of prematurity as compared to twin conception but the outcome is overall better than quadruplet pregnancy. Appropriate doses of Anti D should be administered if Rh negative.

Reduction to a twin pregnancy produces the best chances for the remaining babies. Remainder of pregnancy is managed similar to naturally occurring twins.

Couples may experience feeling of guilt and opportunities for continued counseling should be offered.

Note: *Mean GA to which quadruplets reduced to twin pregnancy may continue is 35 weeks.*

Triplet to twins is 36 weeks.

Pentaplet to twin is 34+5.

Hexaplet to twin is 33+6.

MFPR is done in late first trimester and mainly reduces the number of fetuses. Selective termination mainly concerns the termination of a mal developed fetus after the first trimester.

PAPER 9

1. A 33-year-old woman has had two miscarriages at 8 weeks and one at 14 weeks. She is very anxious and comes to you for advice. Outline the investigations and treatment options for her.
2. A 22-year-old primigravida with no other complications is found to have hemoglobin of 7.8 g/dl at 28 weeks. Discuss her further investigations and management.
3. A 19-year-old primigravida wishes to discuss pain relief during labor. Outline the briefs of your counseling.
4. The routine 18 weeks scan in a 33-year-old primigravida has shown the presence of echogenic bowel. What are the implications of this finding and how will it alter your subsequent care.

1. **A 33-year-old woman has had two miscarriages at 8 weeks and one at 14 weeks. She is very anxious and comes to you for advice. Outline the investigations and treatment options for her.**

Provide lots of supportive care and reassurances. Both partners should preferably be present at time of counseling. Despite the recurrent miscarriages the couple has a 40-50% chance of a healthy live birth without any assistance and treatment. Parental peripheral blood **karyotype** should be performed. 3-5% couples carry a balanced structural abnormality which can result in an unbalanced translocation in the fetus. If an abnormal parental karyotype is identified and the couple is willing to undergo IVF should be referred to a clinical geneticist for genetic counseling, familial chromosomal studies, and prenatal diagnosis in future pregnancies. Cytogenetic analysis of the products of conception should be performed if the next pregnancy fails.

Congenital uterine anomalies may cause second trimester miscarriages and preterm labor. Though the chances of encountering this is less considering the type of history, a **pelvic ultrasound** by skilled personnel should be offered to assess uterine anatomy and morphology. Hysteroscopic septum resection may be helpful in select cases. Routine cervical circlage is not recommended.

Oral glucose tolerance, tests for hyperprolactinemia and thyroid functions are not informative in an asymptomatic woman. Routine progesterone or hCG supplementation is not recommended.

Antithyroid antibodies, and TORCH screening is not helpful in asymptomatic healthy women. Immunotherapy with paternal cell immunisation, donor leucocytes, trophoblast membranes and intravenous immunoglobulin does not improve the live birth rate.

Antiphospholipid antibodies are present in 15% women with recurrent miscarriage. Tests for the presence of **lupus anticoagulant or anticardiolipin antibodies** of IgG and/or IgM class in medium or high titers should be done and repeated again 6 weeks later for the diagnosis of APS. Treatment with low dose aspirin and heparin improves the live birth rate to 70%. Thrombocytopenia and osteopenia should be watched for in women on long-term heparin therapy.

High vaginal swab for the screening of bacterial vaginosis should be offered.

Tests for inherited thrombophilia like APCR, protein C/S and antithrombin III deficiency, and hyperhomocysteinaemia should be performed. Thrombosis in the uteroplacental circulation can cause repeated pregnancy loss. Thromboprophylaxis with heparin may improve pregnancy outcome.

On further conception, further follow-up should be in dedicated early pregnancy units.

2. A 22-year-old primigravida with no other complications is found to have hemoglobin of 7.8 g/dl at 28 weeks. Discuss her further investigations and management.

Hemoglobin levels below 10.5 g/dl are considered abnormal in pregnancy. Iron deficiency is the commonest cause of anemia followed by Folate deficiency. Hemolytic anemia, sickle cell disease, thalassemia and hereditary spherocytosis are other causes for anemia. Ethnicity, family history of anemia and abnormal bleeding should be enquired.

Red cell indices; MCV (mean corpuscular volume), MCH (mean cell hemoglobin) and MCHC (mean cell hemoglobin concentration), serum ferritin, peripheral smear, screening tests for sickle cell and thalassemia trait should be performed.

Low serum ferritin and a microcytic hypochromic anemia suggest iron deficiency anemia. Serum iron less than 12 μmol/l and TIBC saturation less than 15% confirm iron deficiency. Serum ferritin provides assessment into iron stores and is less than 12 μg/l.

Anaemia is associated with low birth weight, preterm delivery and increased blood loss at delivery. Dietary improvements should be suggested under supervision of a dietician. Tea, coffee and chocolate may inhibit iron absorption and should be minimised. Oral Iron supplementation with 100 mg elemental iron should be started and effect of therapy monitored by reticulocyte count 2 weeks later.

Folate deficiency causes a macrocytic anemia with megaloblastic changes in bone marrow. MCV is high and serum and red cell folate are low. 5 mg/day Folate is appropriate for those with established folate deficiency.

Hemoglobin electrophoresis can diagnose sickle cell disease. It causes sickle cell crises, increased miscarriages, IUGR, preterm labor, pre-eclampsia and fetal distress. Infection should be prevented, hypoxia, acidosis, and dehydration need aggressive treatment.

A α and β thalassemia trait and disease may be suspected by finding a low MCV, a low MCH, and a normal MCHC. Diagnosis is confirmed by raised concentrations of HbA_2 and HbF in β thalassemia and by globin chain synthesis studies. Father of the fetus may be offered testing in case of positive result as it may also have implications for all future pregnancies. Oral and parentral iron is contraindicated. Blood transfusions, splenectomy and iron chelation therapy may be required to decrease iron overload in thalassemia major and resistant cases.

If anemia does not respond to oral iron and Folate, IM Folate may be given. Parentral iron may be required if there are problems with compliance or absorption. In such cases, total dose infusion (TDI) should be calculated from body weight and haemoglobin deficiency. It requires sensitivity testing and supervision in hospital. Blood transfusion may be required prior to delivery.

Note: The increased demands for iron are met by increased intestinal absorption. MCV is the first index to become abnormal. Serum iron and TIBC fall in normal pregnancy.

3. A 19-year-old primigravida wishes to discuss pain relief during labor. Outline your approach to counseling the patient.

Presence of a supporting companion during labor and antenatal preparedness of the mother by breathing exercises and antenatal classes helps to decrease fear of labor and decrease the requirement of analgesia.

Non-pharmacological methods like hypnosis, acupuncture, transcutaneous nerve stimulation (TENS), audio analgesia have uncertain efficacy and are unlikely to be used as the sole analgesics during labor.

Nitrous oxide (Entonox-mixture of 50% nitrous oxide and 50% oxygen) is very popular, self administered, intermittent inhalation analgesia. She has to inhale from the mask, at the first feel of contraction. Moderate pain relief is established 20-30 sec later. It is not very successful in women having mask phobia.

Narcotic analgesics like pethidine are given as intramuscular injections (100-150 mg) at the onset of active labor. It has moderate efficacy, with onset of relief within 10-15 min and lasting 3-4 hours. Its depressive effect on fetus is greatest 2-3 hours after maternal administration and least in less than 1 hour or more than 6 hours. It may lead to reduced variability on CTG. The effect may be reversed by naloxone given IM to the fetus.

Pentazocine does not affect the fetal heart rate but may cause hallucinations and no pain relief in upto 40% women.

Patient controlled analgesia involves an infusion of analgesic drug, administered intravenously. The rate of infusion being controlled by a patient controlled pump.

Epidural block involves injection of anaesthetic drug (0.25% bupivacaine and fentanyl) into extradural space in the midline in lateral or sitting position. Adequate circulatory preloading with Hartmann's solution is given to limit any fall in blood pressure. The catheter is usually sited at the onset of active labor and regular top ups are required every 2-3 hours. She will feel the uterine contractions but they are not painful. There is a slight reduction in lower abdominal muscle tone which may decrease maternal expulsive efforts causing a slight prolongation of second stage of labour and increase in operative interference.

Spinal block employs injection of local anaesthetic into subarachnoid space. It is primarily used for second stage procedures like operative vaginal delivery or removal of retained placenta or CS.

Pudendal nerve block is injection of local anaesthetic agents like lignocaine in lateral wall of vagina. Used prior to operative vaginal delivery.

Paracervical nerve block is useful for short-term pain relief during the first stage of labour. Fetal bradycardia and marked vasoconstriction can occur because of inadvertent administration in uterine artery.

Local infiltration of perineum by lignocaine is effective in reducing the pain due to episiotomy.

Information leaflets and contact addresses of hospital antenatal classes should be provided to her.

Note: During the first stage of labor, nerves from T_{10}-L_1 should be blocked and S_2-S_5 during the second stage.

Epidural space is between dura mater and bony vertebral canal bound by ligamentum flavum and posterior ligament of the vertebrae.

Absolute contraindications of epidural include—refused maternal permission, sepsis in lumbosacral region, conditions predisposing to caugulopathy (severe pre- eclampsia, placental abruption, prolonged retention of products of conception, and thrombocytopenia), use of anticoagulants (except LMWH), severe maternal hypotension and active substantial hemorrhage. Progressive neurological disease is a relative contraindication.

Complications of epidural are: Bloody tap, dural punctures (causing headaches), sympathetic block (causing fall in blood pressure- give 5 mg ephedrine if fall is more than 20 mm Hg), total spinal block (causing cardiovascular and respiratory collapse) and partial blocks.

4. **The routine 18 weeks scan in a 33-year-old primigravida has shown the presence of echogenic bowel. What are the implications of this finding and how will it alter your subsequent care.**

- Fetal bowel is considered hyperechogenic when its echogenicity is grossly similar to or greater than that of surrounding bone (fetal iliac crest) regardless of the shape of the echogenic mass in the same machine settings.
- It can be a physiological variant in 67% cases.
- It may be associated with an increased risk of cystic fibrosis, meconium ileus, cytomegalovirus (CMV) infection, adverse fetal outcome such as intrauterine growth restriction and fetal death. It is considered a soft marker for fetal trisomy 21.
- Finding a hyperechogenic bowel on ultrasound therefore warrants careful investigations.
- Blood samples from mother and father should be tested for DNA mutation analysis for cystic fibrosis. CMV IgM should be tested in maternal blood. Amniocentesis for fetal karyotyping and detection of aneuploidies should be offered in the presence of other soft markers or suspicious serum screening. In the absence of paternal blood samples, DNA mutation analysis for cystic fibrosis can be done from amniotic fluid. Risks associated with amniocentesis should be explained to the mother.
- High levels of parental anxiety associated with such findings should be acknowledged and expert counseling arranged for if so desired.
- Termination of pregnancy option may be offered if fetus is found to be affected by Down's syndrome or cystic fibrosis.
- Even in the absence of any detectable abnormality, remainder of the pregnancy should be supervised by 3-4 weekly scans for early detection of growth restriction. Careful search for other ultrasonographic anomalies should be made and if required, woman may be referred to a center of expertise for the same.
- Infant may be subjected to immunoreactive trypsin assay and sweat testing to confirm the absence of cystic fibrosis if no testing has been done in parents.

Note: Δ F 508 is the commonest mutation causing cystic fibrosis in UK white population.

Soft markers are minor ultrasonographic features which may be present in normal fetuses, but have been found in association with abnormal karyotypes.

Echogenic bowel is easily confused with calcifications associated with fetal infection, bowel obstruction/perforation/meconium peritonitis.

Maternal age more than 35 years is an independent risk factor and karyotyping should be offered to such women with echogenic bowel in the absence of any other abnormality.

PAPER 10

1. A 30-year-old parous woman at 28 weeks of pregnancy presents at A&E with high grade fever and loin pain. Her urine dipstick test for nitrites is positive. How will you manage her?
2. A 31-year-old woman attends for booking visit at 26 weeks. Shortly before becoming pregnant her cervical smear showed severe dyskaryosis. Discuss management of her abnormal smear and possible implications for pregnancy.
3. Discuss the various tests that can be used to screen the presence of Down's syndrome in pregnancy.
4. During routine antenatal visit a 26-year-old parous woman reveals that she developed severe depression after her last child birth. Outline your approach to wards her.

1. **A 30-year-old parous woman at 28 weeks of pregnancy presents at A&E with high grade fever and loin pain. Her urine dipstick test for nitrites is positive. How will you manage her?**

She should be hospitalised. The most likely diagnosis is pyelonephritis. Ascertain a history of previous such episodes. Women with diabetes and on steroid therapy are more vulnerable to developing pyelonephritis.

Maternal pulse, temperature, blood pressure, intake and urinary output record should be monitored. Hypotension and tachycardia are ominous signs.

Full blood count, serum urea, creatinine, electrolytes, 24 hours creatinine clearance, a mid-stream urine sample (MSU) for culture and blood cultures should be sent.

Ultrasound KUB to exclude hydronephrosis, congenital abnormalities and calculi should be done. Chest X-ray with abdominal shield should be done to exclude pneumonia if there is tachypnoea or chest signs.

IV antibiotics should be commenced without waiting for the culture results. IV amoxi-clav (1g 6 h) or cephalosporin's (cefuroxime-750 mg 8 h) are usually the first choice. In allergic /resistant cases an amino glycoside such as gentamicin may be added. IV antibiotics should be continued till the patient is afebrile for 24 hours. After that oral preparations should be continued for at least 2 weeks.

Appropriate intravenous fluids to maintain urinary output >30 ml/hour should be given. Antiemetics may be required initially if vomiting is severe. Paracetamol should be used to reduce pyrexia.

Renal functions and blood chemistry should be reassessed after 48 hours and then periodically depending on severity. Multidisciplinary approach with involvement of nephrologists and urologists is required if there is no clinical improvement within 72 hours.

One in four women have a transient but significant decline in renal and hematological parameters suggested by thrombocytopenia, anemia, DIC, hemolysis, perinephric abscess, septicemic shock and ARDS.

Risk of preterm delivery and low birth weight babies increase significantly. Antenatal steroids should be added and fetal well-being monitored periodically by NST and ultrasound studies.

She can be discharged if she has been afebrile for 24-48 hours. She should be advised to increase her oral intake of clear fluids. Follow-up antenatal visit should be arranged after 3 weeks and repeat urine culture taken.

Postpartum intravenous urography should be offered to women having history of recurrent UTI in pregnancy.

Note: *4-7% pregnant women have asymptomatic bacteriuria, of whom up to 40% will develop symptomatic urinary tract infection in pregnancy.*

Two percent develop pyelonephritis.

80-90% of bacteriuria is due to E. coli and is related to sexual intercourse related ascending infection from perineum.

Significant bacteriuria occurs with colony counts more than 10^5/ml of MSU specimen.

Screening and treatment of asymptomatic bacteriuria will prevent 70% of all cases of pyelonephritis.

2. **A 31-year-old woman attends for antepartum visit at 26 weeks. Shortly before becoming pregnant her cervical smear showed severe dyskaryosis. Discuss management of her abnormal smear and possible implications for pregnancy.**

Progressive potential of severe dyskaryosis is 20% at 10 years and 80-90% women will have CIN II-III at the time of diagnosis of an abnormal cytological smear is the same as in non-pregnant women. She should be urgently referred for colposcopy and seen within 4 weeks. Further management depends on colposcopic findings.

If invasion is suspected, directed biopsy may be required for histo-pathological confirmation. Colposcopically directed punch biopsies are safe and are 99% accurate in pregnancy. Associated bleeding due to pregnancy induced hyperemia can usually be controlled by vaginal packing, silver nitrate or haemostatic sutures. If biopsy confirms invasion, an MRI should be done to see the extent of lesion, and deliver by cesarean section at 34 weeks after a course of steroids. If biopsy shows a non invasive lesion (CIN I, II, III) treatment should be deferred till after delivery.

If after initial colposcopic examination, invasion is not suspected, woman is followed up 6-12 weeks after delivery for a "See and treat policy". If any suspicious findings are present after colposcopy, a repeat biopsy is taken otherwise she is kept under follow-up. If CIN I is identified on this biopsy, simply repeating the cervical smears after 6 months is adequate. If repeat smear shows the abnormality, ablative methods like cryotherapy and cold coagulation or laser vaporization may be used in such women.

If CIN II or III is identified, woman must be allowed to make an informed decision regarding the mode of treatment. Excisional methods like LLETZ (large loop excision of transformation zone), NETZ (needle diathermy excision) are the mainstay of treatment. Even after adequate treatment 5% women will have recurrence within 2 years. Annual cytological follow-up should be done for at least 10 years.

Note: All women between the ages of 25 and 49 should have cervical screening with Pap smear every 3 years, and between 50-64 years, every 5 years. The results should normally be made available in writing from the GP within 6 weeks.

Cancer of the cervix is the second most common cancer worldwide, after cancer breast in women under 35 years.

3. Discuss the various tests that can be used to screen the presence of Down's syndrome in pregnancy.

The aim of antenatal screening for Down's syndrome (DS) is to offer women, during pregnancy, a screening test which can identify those women at higher risk of having an affected child. The group at increased risk is then offered diagnostic tests.

To ensure uniformity and consistency in reporting, a risk cutoff of 1 in 250 at term has been adopted. All screening tests take maternal age into account.

UK Down's syndrome screening program has adopted a new benchmark for screening tests, to be achieved by 1st April 2007, i.e. tests should have a detection rate (DR) of at least 75% with a false positive rate (FPR) of <3%. SURUSS provided the required evidence leading to this policy.

Integrated test: Best performance test provided good quality nuchal translucency (NT) measurement is available and woman is ready to wait until the 2nd trimester for results. It integrates NT +PAPP-A (pregnancy associated plasma protein A) measured at 10 completed weeks and Quadruple test done at 14-20 weeks into a single test result. At 85% DR, the FPR is only 1.2%. This ensures higher safety by decreasing rate of loss of unaffected fetuses. Due to lowest FPR, it is cost effective.

Serum integrated test: It is potentially the best if NT measurements are not available. Uses only serum markers: PAPP-A at 10 weeks +Quadruple test at 14-20 weeks.

At 85% DR it has a FPR of 2.7%.

Combined test: It is for women who require screening in first trimester and understand the implications of doing so. Combines NT measurement +β hCG+PAPP-A at 10 weeks.

At 85%DR the FPR is 6.1%.

Quadruple test: Second trimester test for women who attend late.

Measures Alpha-fetoprotein (AFP) + unconjugated estriol+ β hCG + inhibin-A.

At 85% DR it has FPR of 6.2%.

Triple test: Second trimester test. Measures AFP+μ E_3 +β hCG at 14-20 weeks.

At DR of 85%, FPR is 9.3%.

Double test: Second trimester test. Measures AFP+ β hCG. FPR is 13.1%.

Nuchal translucency measurement: Done at 11-13 completed weeks and has FPR of 20% if used alone.

Before measuring the serum levels of markers, gestational age should be assessed accurately. Most accurate dating is by an early dating scan done between 8-12 weeks + 6 days.

Screening performance of first trimester and second trimester tests is similar. Screening in individual trimesters is much less effective than integrating serial measurements from both trimesters into a single test.

SURUSS does not support retaining double/triple test/NT measurements on their own as each would lead to many more invasive diagnostic tests without increasing the proportion of DS pregnancies detected.

Written information must be given and discussed with all pregnant women prior to screening procedure, to enable them to make an informed choice.

Note: The earlier performance standard for the tests was DR>60% with FPR 5% or less to be achieved by April 2005.

SURUSS: First and second trimester antenatal screening for Down's syndrome; the results of serum, urine and ultrasound screening study.

In DS pregnancy, μE_3 and AFP are lower while hCG, PAPP-A and inhibin A are elevated.

95% of non-disjunction trisomy 21 is maternal in origin and the risk increases with increase in maternal age. Likelihood of fetus with DS at 35 years is 1:140, at 40 years 1:45, at 45 years 1:15.

Translocation trisomy (inherited/*de novo*) is not associated with maternal age.

Cost to UK NHS is estimated to be £ 15,300 per affected pregnancy detected by integrated test, £16,800 by quadruple test, and £ 19,000 by combined test.

4. During routine antenatal visit a 26-year-old parous woman reveals that she developed severe depression after the birth of her last child. Outline your approach to wards her.

This woman should be considered high risk for developing depression in the postpartum period as a previous episode is an indicator and risk factor for the same.

Assess her current status by eliciting detailed past and family psychiatric history, current medications, social and financial support. Her relationship with her parents, partner and other children should be explored. Encourage her to reveal any stressful life events regarding her occupation, finances, loss in the family or friends. Any suicidal thoughts or tendency for self harm should be enquired directly.

Symptoms of depression like increased anxiety, weepiness, insomnia, decreased self worth and poor self-esteem should be enquired. Antenatal depression increases her chances of having postpartum depression.

Explanation and reassurance about her condition should be provided sympathetically. One in ten women experience some form of postnatal depressive illness.

Multidisciplinary approach by early referral to psychiatrist and, clinical psychologist for assessment should be adopted. Community based midwife and general practitioner should be involved in her care during the postnatal period. She should be advised to get in touch with the local health visitor and the importance of psychological support should be emphasized to the partner. Cognitive behavior therapy should be offered.

Contact numbers of voluntary support organizations like MAMA (Meet a Mum), and the association for post natal illness should be provided to her.

If symptomatic, consideration should be given to start psychotropic drugs. Lithium is contraindicated in first trimester and cardiac scan should be offered at 22 weeks if she continues to take lithium. Tricyclic antidepressants are safe to use during pregnancy.

Vigilance should be maintained to look for any abnormal behavior, abnormal concerns about baby or self, in the postnatal period. In severe cases she should be transferred to dedicated mother and baby units along with the infant. Electroconvulsive therapy (ECT) is not contraindicated for severe cases. Care should be taken to ensure baby's safety.

Prophylaxis with antidepressants can be considered in the postnatal period but as the peak incidence is around 6 weeks postpartum long-term community based care should be arranged.

Encourage breastfeeding as it enhances woman's self image. If she is on psychotropic medication infant should be watched for signs of toxicity. Continue antidepressants for at least 6 months. Most tricyclics and sertraline are safe during lactation. Individual assessment regarding risk vs. benefit of breastfeeding should be made after discussion with the woman.

Risk of recurrence depends on severity of depression and varies from 25-50%.

Note:

Incidence of maternity blues—50%

Incidence of postnatal depression—10-15%

Incidence of puerperal psychosis—0.2%

According to DSM -1V criteria, postpartum depression is diagnosed when the woman experiences at least 5 of the following criteria for over 2 weeks;

Depressed mood, anhedonia, significant changes in weight or appetite, insomnia or hypersomnia, psychomotor agitation or retardation, fatigue, inappropriate guilt or feeling of worthlessness, impaired concentration or indecisiveness and recurrent thoughts of death or suicide.

PAPER 11

1. A 30-year-old primigravida presents at 32 weeks' gestation with generalized itching but no skin rash. How will you confirm the diagnosis and manage the remainder of her pregnancy?
2. Discuss the management of a twin pregnancy complicated by antenatal demise of one of the fetuses diagnosed at 30 weeks.
3. A 32-year-old woman has been referred to you by the GP with a random blood sugar of 8.3 mmol/l. She is currently 18 weeks pregnant and has no history of diabetes mellitus before. How will you manage her pregnancy.
4. A 20-year-old has tested positive for HIV during her booking investigations. How will you manage the rest of her pregnancy?

1. A 30-year-old primigravida presents at 32 weeks' gestation with generalized itching but no skin rash. How will you confirm the diagnosis and manage the remainder of her pregnancy?

The most likely diagnosis is obstetric cholestasis (OC or intrahepatic cholestasis of pregnancy). It is a diagnosis of exclusion. A history of onset of pruritis from second trimester onwards in the absence of rash and altered liver functions is significant. Family history may be found in one-third of the cases. Sleep deprivation, Jaundice, (pale stools and dark urine) and steatorrhoea may be associated symptoms.

Liver function tests may reveal mild increase in bilirubin, alkaline phosphatase, gamma-glutamyl transpeptide and total bile acids. There is usually a 2-3 fold increase in transaminases (ALT being most sensitive) and up to 100-fold increase in primary bile acids (cholic acid and chenodeoxycholic acid). Pregnancy specific range for transaminases should be taken for reference. In the presence of normal bile salt levels, other hepatic pathology should be looked for. In the presence of persistent pruritis and normal liver function, the tests should be repeated weekly.

Liver ultrasound and viral serology (hepatitis A, B, C, EBV, and CMV) should be done to exclude other causes of deranged liver functions and itching.

Once a diagnosis of OC is made the woman should be counseled concerning the fetal risks like possible preterm delivery, meconium stained liquor, intrapartum fetal distress, intrauterine fetal death and fetal intracranial hemorrhages. Fetal well being should be monitored closely by 3 weekly ultrasound scans to check fetal growth, liquor volume, and Doppler umbilical artery blood flow studies.

Mother is more prone to get vitamin K mal absorption. Tab vitamin K 10 g oral every day should be commenced after 36 weeks and continued till delivery.

Liver function tests and prothrombin time should be checked weekly.

Frequency of antenatal visits should be determined by the severity of condition.

Cool baths, bicarbonate washes and topical emollients are helpful in mild cases. Chlorpheniramine at bed time may help to relieve pruritis. Ursodeoxycholic acid to decrease the total bile acid levels is not licensed for use in pregnancy.

Cholestiramine may be effective in some women. S-adenosylmethionine (SAM), guar gum, and activated charcoal have no role.

Offer to deliver her at 38 weeks as risk of fetal death may increase after 36 weeks. If condition aggravates, antenatal steroids should be given before 34 weeks. Risk of induction and possible cesarean section should be explained to the mother.

Labor should be closely monitored by electronic fetal monitoring and precautions taken to prevent PPH. Neonate should receive injection vitamin K at birth.

After delivery, pruritis may take 1-2 weeks for resolution. Repeat LFT's after 10-14 days to check resolution. If required biliary tract ultrasound for gallstones should be performed. Risk of recurrence in subsequent pregnancies is high 50-60%. Standard estrogen containing oral contraceptives should be avoided but low dose preparations may be advised under supervision.

Note: Incidence of OC is higher in women of Asian origin especially Indian and Pakistani women. In pregnancy upper limit of bilirubin and gamma glutamyltransferase is 15-20% lower.

2. Discuss the management of a twin pregnancy complicated by antenatal demise of one of the fetuses diagnosed at 30 weeks.

The chorionicity of the twins should have been determined by early ultrasound scanning. In monochorionic pregnancies, the mortality and morbidity of surviving twin is greatly increased. One in four fetuses will have neurological damage, including cerebral palsy, porencephaly, hydrocephalus and cerebral infarction. Renal cortical necrosis may occur. Dichorionic pregnancies will have a better prognosis as communicating vessels are very uncommon.

Offer bereavement counseling to the mother and family.

DIC in the mother can be a complication *in utero* demise and immediate and weekly coagulation studies should be carried out.

Investigations to check uteroplacental insufficiency and hostile uterine environment should be carried out as they could be a threat to the surviving twin as well.

The surviving twin should be serially assessed by using cardiotocography and ultrasound (biophysical profile, biometry).

Antenatal corticosteroids should be given to mother to prevent neonatal respiratory distress in surviving twin in case of premature delivery.

The psychological status of woman and her preferences should be taken into account before deciding about the time of delivery. Risks of prematurity versus the risk of *in utero* damage must be balanced. Expectant management may be adopted especially when >24 hours have elapsed since the event. Feto fetal transfusion and the ischemic injury to the surviving twin is an acute event. Cesarean section is generally the preferred route if preterm delivery is indicated. Delivery may be delayed up to 37 weeks in dichorionic pregnancy in the absence of any maternal or fetal compromise.

After delivery the newborn should be assessed by cranial ultrasound and MRI in case of any abnormality. Baby may require prolonged neurodevelopmental follow-up by pediatricians.

GP and social worker should be informed at the time of discharge to offer extended support and counseling to the couple.

3. **A 32-year-old woman has been referred to you by the GP with a random blood sugar of 8.3 mmol/l. She is currently 18 weeks pregnant and has no history of diabetes mellitus before. How will you manage her pregnancy.**

History of previous poor obstetrical outcome, (macrosomia, unexplained still birth), positive family history of diabetes increases her likelihood of gestational diabetes (GDM). Enquiries should be made regarding the relation of meals with the test as one random sample on its own is suggestive but not sufficient for diagnosis of diabetes and formal 2 hours oral GTT should be done after 8 hours of fasting followed by 75 gm glucose load. Further management depends on the result of O-GTT and she should be classified as normal, impaired GTT or gestational diabetes mellitus (GDM). If normal, pregnancy should procced as per protocol and GTT should be repeated at 28-30 weeks of gestation and the situation reviewed.

Investigations: Blood pressure and body mass index should be noted. glycosylated hemoglobin (HbA1$_c$), routine pregnancy investigations and urinalysis should be performed in all patients. Gestational age should be accurately calculated from first trimester sonar. Offer screening for neural tube defects and Down's syndrome.

If she has mild degrees of impaired glucose tolerance, she should be reassured as the perinatal outcome is similar to that in healthy population. A timed random glucose sample and urine for glycosuria should be checked at each antenatal visit. Life style and dietary modifications should be suggested. Diet with reduced fat, increased fiber and regulated carbohydrate intake of low glycemic index should be stressed. She should omit intake of large quantities of high calorie foods and snacks, carbonated drinks, and fresh orange juice. Total intake should be spread between 3 main meals and 3 snacks. Usually such women achieve good control with dietary modification, exercise, with or without low dose insulin.

If she is classified as GDM, a multidisciplinary team should be involved in her care. Detailed anomaly scan should be performed at 18-20 weeks and cardiac scan should be considered at 24 weeks. Serial scans may be required to assess fetal growth and liquor volume. Strict compliance with diebetic diet should be advised.

A baseline 24 hours blood sugar profile should be done and repeated serially depending on the severity. Persistent postprandial hyperglycemia (> 7.5-8 mmol/l) or fasting hyperglycemia (> 5.5 mmol/l) despite compliance with diet for a week are indications for introduction of insulin therapy. Dietary modifications should continue till term in addition to insulin.

She should be encouraged to monitor her own blood sugar at home (HBGM) with glucometers, the frequency of monitoring being proportional to derangement in blood sugar. Human actrapid insulin should be preferred with its dose and frequency being adjusted by postprandial values.

Elective cesarean section may be considered in the presence of mal-presentations, an estimated fetal weight in excess of 4.5 kg, or a history of previous cesarean section.

Continue pregnancy till term if good control of diabetes is achieved. Each case should be assessed individually regarding time of induction, if required. Routine inductions at 38 weeks and waiting till 41 weeks have similar CS and shoulder dystocia rates.

Adequate labor analgesia (epidural) should be considered to avoid catecholamine associated hyperglycemia. Labor should be carefully supervised with partograms and experienced midwifery staff.

Women with impaired GTT either do not require insulin during labor or small doses are given using a sliding scale. Those on larger doses of insulin should be managed by insulin infusions as per the labor ward protocol.

Encourage breastfeeding after delivery. Progesterone only pills, barriers and low dose estrogen pills can be prescribed for contraception. Offer her GTT with 75 gm glucose within 6 weeks to 3 months of delivery to assess her status. She should be made aware of the long-term risk of developing NIDDM associated with GDM. Recurrence rate in next pregnancy can be minimized by achieving ideal BMI prior to conception.

Note: Women with GDM have 50% risk of developing NIDDM within 10-15 years. Insulin and glucagons do not cross placenta. There is no increase in brain size in macrosomic fetuses. AFP, E_3, and hCG values are all lower in diabetics.

GDM is diagnosed if:

1. After 50 gm glucose load orally, blood sugar level after 1 hour is > 7.8 mmol/l.
2. Fasting blood glucose level is > 6.0 mmol/l and 2 hours postprandial value is >9.0 mmol/l (adopted by UK Task force on diabetes) but local guidelines should be followed for treatment purposes.

3. The WHO proposes the following criteria after 75 g oral GTT

	Normal	Impaired	Frank diabetes
Fasting	< 6 mmol/l	6- 7.9 mmol/l	≥ 8 mmol/l and/or
2 hours PP	<9 mmol/l	9-10.9 mmol/l	≥ 11.1 mmol/l

Target plasma glucose levels in pregnancy are:

Before breakfast	69-90 mg/dl or 4-5 mmol/l
Before lunch, dinner	60-105 mg/dl or 4- 6 mmol/l
After meals	= 120 mg/dl or less than 6.8 mmol/l
2 AM to 6 AM	> 60 mg/dl or more than 4 mmol/l

For frank diabetics and those requiring high doses of insulin in antenatal period infusions of human actrapid insulin 10 units in 100 ml of normal saline should be started at 10 ml/hr using a micro drip set. Blood sugar should be checked hourly in the other arm. If blood sugar is between 4-6 mmol/l continue the same dose of insulin. If <4 mmol, halve the rate of infusion and if >6 mmol then double the rate of insulin infusion till optimum sugar levels are achieved. Halve the rate of insulin infusion after delivery. In the other arm she should constantly receive 100 ml/hr of 10% dextrose.

18 mg = 1mmol of glucose.

4. A 20-year-old has tested positive for HIV during her booking investigations. How will you manage the rest of her pregnancy?

She should be informed of her HIV result in person, by an appropriately trained health professional. Information leaflets and all information about her subsequent care should be imparted in a non-judgmental manner.

Reassure her repeatedly that her confidentiality will be respected. However, all health professionals involved in her care should be aware of her diagnosis. She should be encouraged to inform her seropositive status to her partner but no information should be revealed to people (relatives) who are not at risk of acquiring infection.

Termination of pregnancy is an option if the women so desires.

She should be managed by a multidisciplinary team including an HIV physician, an obstetrician, midwife, pediatrician, psychiatric team and support groups. The case should be reported to National study of HIV in pregnancy and childhood at RCOG.

Baseline investigations like complete blood counts including CD4-T lymphocyte count, maternal plasma viral load, serum urea, electrolytes, liver enzymes, blood glucose and lactates should be done and repeated monthly. She should be screened for inflammatory genital infections (*Chlamydia, gonorrhea*, bacterial vaginosis) as soon as possible in pregnancy and at 28 weeks. Screening for syphilis, hepatitis B, and HCV should be offered.

Routine pregnancy investigations, detailed ultrasound for fetal anomalies and Down's syndrome screening should be offered.

Antepartum: She should be informed that interventions such as antiretroviral therapy, elective cesarean section and avoidance of breastfeeding can reduce the incidence of vertical transmission from 25-30% to less than 2%.

Women having low plasma viral load and CD4 –T lymphocyte count $> 350 \times 10^6/l$ require antiretroviral therapy to decrease risk of vertical transmission. Short term antiretroviral therapy (START) from 28-32 weeks (oral Ziduvudine 100 mg 5 times a day) should be started and continued intrapartum. If she is at high risk for preterm delivery (uterine over distension, previous history) therapy should be commenced earlier to achieve undetectable plasma viral load by delivery. Prophylactic steroids to enhance lung maturity should be given if required.

Women having symptomatic HIV infection, or low CD4 counts should be advised to commence highly active retroviral therapy (HAART) from 14-34 weeks and continued till after delivery. Optimal drug and dose regimen, decision to start, modify or stop retroviral therapy should be determined by an HIV physician in close liaison with the obstetrician and pediatrician.

Drug toxicities include cholestasis, GI upsets, fatigue, fever, hepatotoxicity, rashes, glucose intolerance, diabetes, lactic acidosis and mild anemia. If CD4 counts are $<200 \times 10^6/l$ prophylaxis against *Pneumocystis carinii* pneumonia infection should be given by administering cotrimoxazole and folic acid.

Intrapartum: She should be offered elective cesarean section at 38 weeks. Ziduvudine infusion should be started 4 hours prior to skin incision and continued till umbilical cord is clamped. Prophylactic antibiotics should be given to decrease infective morbidity.

Women who prefer to avoid cesarean section should have their membranes left intact for as long as possible. Fetal scalp electrodes and scalp sampling should be avoided. Ziduvudine infusion (or HAART) should be commenced at onset of labor and continued till cord is clamped. HIV infection per se is not an indication for electronic fetal monitoring.

Maternal serum samples should be taken for viral loads at delivery. Cord should be clamped as soon as possible and baby should be given bath immediately after birth.

Postpartum: She should be advised not to breastfeed the baby as it increases perinatal transmission. Infant should be treated with antiretroviral drugs for 4 to 6 weeks. Polymerase chain reaction (PCR) should be done at birth, 3 weeks, 6 weeks and 6 months to detect infant viral infection.

Appropriate contraception and use of barriers should be promoted at all times.

Note: HIV is a human retrovirus with double stranded DNA. Zidovudine; the commonest medicine in use inhibits chain elongation of viral DNA by selectively inhibiting RNA dependent DNA polymerase (viral reverse transcriptase).

Over 80% of mother to child (vertical) transmission occurs late in the 3rd trimester, during labor and at delivery with less than 2% transmission during 1st and 2nd trimesters. Low antenatal CD4-T lymphocyte counts ($< 350 \times 10^6/l$), high maternal plasma viral loads ($>20,000$ copies/ml), vaginal delivery, duration of membrane rupture >4 hours, chorioamnionitis and preterm labor are associated with increased risk of transmission.

Breastfeeding doubles the risk of vertical transmission from 14 to 28%.

PAPER 12

1. Compare and contrast the methods used for invasive prenatal diagnosis.
2. A 30-year-old woman has just had an unexplained stillbirth. You are the SpR on duty and have to take consent for postmortem of the baby. What are the issues involved?
3. 34-year-old woman on thyroxine supplements for hypothyroidism comes to you for advice. She is asymptomatic at present and wishes to start her family. How will you counsel her?
4. A multigravid woman has been referred to you as the midwife suspects the fetus to be small for dates. She is currently 28 weeks pregnant and has had 2 previous normal deliveries with normal outcome. Discuss her management.

ompare and contrast the methods used for invasive prenatal
diagnosis.

Chorionic villous sampling (CVS) is the aspiration of chorion frondosum (placenta) between 9-13 weeks of pregnancy. The primary indication is early exclusion of maternal age related aneuploidy and previous history of an aneuploid fetus.

It can be performed by transvaginal, transabdominal, or transcervical route under direct ultrasound control.

Advantages: Rapid; result available within 72 hours. Safer as compared to early amniocentesis.

More acceptable in high risk women who have already experienced a late termination of pregnancy due to aneuploidy in a previous pregnancy.

Complications: As compared to second trimester amniocentesis a higher number of repeat procedures may be required for diagnosis; miscarriage rate is higher (1-2%) and a higher incidence of limb reduction defects (0.05% if performed after 9 weeks to-0.3%before 9 weeks).

Contamination of chorionic cell cultures with maternal cells can cause a false negative diagnosis. There is 1% risk of Mosaicism (8 times higher than amniocentesis) and other placental variants.

Placental biopsy is akin to CVS but is performed in the second trimester where a large amount of DNA or rapid karyotype is required. It is the method of choice for second trimester diagnosis of monogenic disorders. Direct chromosomal preparations can be made from sample and result can be available within 24 hours. It is only performed transabdominally. Risk of fetomaternal hemorrhage and late termination of pregnancy are in addition to risks of CVS.

Amniocentesis is removal of amniotic fluid for karyotyping. It is the commonest invasive prenatal diagnostic procedure performed in UK and has high patient acceptability.

It is performed transabdominally between 15-18 weeks under ultrasound guidance. 'Early' amniocentesis is performed before 15 weeks; has higher complication rate and fetal talipes.

A rapid test result (PCR) is available within 72 hours for Down's syndrome and a few aneuploidies but a negative culture report takes 2-3 weeks. About 0.5% of cultures fail and maternal contamination leads to diagnostic difficulties in <0.2%.

Complications; Fetal loss (0.5-1% risk), preterm labor and delivery, lung hypoplasia, respiratory distress, postural limb deformities, fetal trauma by needle, risk of alloimmunisation in rheuses negative women (15%), bloody tap (0.5%).

Cordocentesis: Removal of fetal blood from umbilical cord vessels. Performed transabdominally after 18 weeks. Used for diagnosis of chromosomal abnormalities (fetal malformation or IUGR), single gene defect like hemoglobinopathies, severity of fetal anemia, thrombocytopenia, acidosis and fetal infection. Site of blood withdrawal could be from placental umbilical cord insertion (commonest), fetal heart or fetal intrahepatic vessels.

Procedure related loss varies from 1-2% and vary according to operator expertise.

Complications include; bleeding/hematoma at puncture site, reflex fetal bradycardia, infection, PPROM, placental abruption, preterm labor, and fetal death. Maternal risk of alloimmunisation, chorioamnionitis, trauma, emergency CS, and psychological effects of fetal loss.

Results are available in 48-72 hours and it can only be performed in specialized fetomaternal medicine units. It is difficult to perform and has a long learning curve.

Fetoscopy: It involves visualization of fetal anatomical defects by passing a telescope through the fetus. With the advent of safer techniques and high fetal losses associated with the procedure it is no longer used.

2. A 30-year-old woman has just had an unexplained stillbirth. You are the SpR on duty and have to take consent for postmortem of the baby. What are the issues involved?

The women should be handled sympathetically and discussions should preferably take place with both the partners together. A written informed consent from the mother is required for the procedure. Standard perinatal autopsy request and report forms should be filled.

Acknowledge that discussions about autopsy are acutely distressful following bereavement and refusal for the same is her right in case of personal or religious objections.

She should be informed that autopsy may confirm clinical diagnosis, reveal the cause of death, reveal structural anomalies of relevance to the risk of recurrence, provide an estimate to the time of death, identify chronic intrauterine disease (infection, brain damage, etc.) and give information on the complications of treatment. It may be difficult, if not impossible, to advise on the risk of recurrence in a future pregnancy in the absence of autopsy. Even a negative or normal autopsy report is of significance and in some cases no abnormality may be revealed. Sometimes despite tests it is not possible to know the exact cause of death.

Consent is required for:

1. Postmortem examination and tissue retention of small samples for histopathological diagnosis. To investigate the molecular basis of unexplained death, fetal DNA should be stored to detect later, the disorders which may later be shown to have genetic basis. DNA extraction requires considerable workload and storage of small amount of fetal tissue is more practical.

2. Use of material (histopathological slides) for teaching, research and possible tissue retention for treatment of others.

3. Organ retention; especially brain and heart for diagnosis of congenital disorders. Whenever possible organs are reunited with body prior to burial or cremation. When it is not possible, parents can choose either to make their own arrangements or leave it to the hospital to dispose of the organs after investigations have been completed.

Every hospital should have written guidelines for external and radiological examination and for maternal and neonatal investigations in case of perinatal death. Use of fetal tissues and organs can only be carried out if the hospital conforms to Polkinghorne guidelines.

Parents who decline perinatal autopsy should be offered limited autopsy. This includes external examination, tissue needle biopsy, body cavity aspiration, imaging (X-ray, ultrasound, MRI), targeted open tissue biopsy and placental biopsy. Post stillbirth karyotyping has high failure rate. Multiple samples should be collected, usually from placenta and full thickness skin biopsies. Specific consent for each component should be taken. It must be stressed that these techniques remain inferior alternatives to full postmortem with histopathology.

Bodies need to be transported from place of delivery/death to a regional center for specialist autopsy by a perinatal pathologist. Consent should be taken for this transfer. She should be informed about means of transport and when the body will be returned. Written procedures for handling, receipt and return of bodies should exist. Inform the mother that the case will be taken up for discussion at perinatal mortality meeting.

Information leaflet should be provided to the parents explaining the purpose of an autopsy, benefits of tissue and organ retention and rights of parents to grant or withhold their agreement. CESDI document "Guide to the postmortem examination: Brief notes for parents and families who have lost a baby in pregnancy and infancy" should be recommended.

- Cause of death
- reveal structural anomalies
- identify chrom in to autu disceon (infection, brain damage etc)
= Chance f recurence.

Maternal

fetal.

3. **34-year-old woman on thyroxine supplements for hypothyroidism comes to you for advice. She is asymptomatic at present and wishes to start her family. How will you counsel her?**

The commonest causes of hypothyroidism in women are iodine deficiency and autoimmune thyroiditis. Enquiries regarding duration, dosage, type of supplement being taken and any pertinent symptoms should be made.

Baseline thyroid functions and drug levels should be measured and pregnancy deferred till medical optimization is achieved. General advice regarding rubella status, cigarette smoking, cervical screening and folic acid supplementation should be given.

If she is already on adequate replacement therapy, reassurance should be offered, as maternal and fetal outcome is usually good and unaffected by the hypothyroidism.

Untreated hypothyroidism may be associated with infertility, an increased rate of miscarriage, anemia, pre-eclampsia, low birth weight infants, prematurity, still birth and fetal loss.

Even subclinical hypothyroidism may be associated with reduced intelligence quotient and neurodevelopmental delay in the offspring. Severe deficiency may cause permanent brain damage and neurological cretinism in the child.

Very little thyroxine crosses the placenta and the fetus is not at risk of thyrotoxicosis from maternal thyroxine replacement therapy. Neonatal hypothyroidism may rarely result from transplacental passage of TSH receptor blocking antibodies.

Pregnancy itself has no effect on disease progression. Early pregnancy is characterized by relative hyperthyroidism whereas there is a small decline in T_3 and T_4 levels in the second and third trimesters but all parameters remain within the normal range. If she is euthyroid at the beginning of pregnancy, usually no further increments in her thyroxine doses are required during pregnancy or in the puerperium.

Free T_4 (low), TSH (high), thyroid auto antibodies (may be present) Complete blood counts, (normocytic anemia) lipid profile (hyperlipedemia), liver function (deranged) and any specific investigations regarding the cause of hypothyroidism may be done at booking visit.

Hypothyroidism may be associated with other autoimmune disorders like insulin dependent diabetes mellitus, pernicious anemia and vitiligo. Search and appropriate investigations to rule out the same should be carried out. Thyroid functions should be done during the first trimester and at least once during each trimester to ensure adequate replacement. Following any adjustment in thyroxine dose, thyroid unction should be checked after 4-6 weeks. Any increments in doses should be made cautiously in case of heart disease.

Drugs like iron supplements and antacids containing aluminium hydroxide interfere with thyroxine absorption and should be taken at different times.

No specific plans are needed for labor or delivery if she is adequately controlled.

One in ten women will have residual postpartum dysfunction with an initial hyperthyroidism which may last for 2-3 months postpartum, followed by hypothyroidism. Management during initial puerperium should be symptomatic and 4 weekly assessment of antimicrosomal antibody titers.

Note: Placenta is freely permeable to TRH, TSH autoantibodies and iodine, not to TSH and thyroxine. Isolated thyroid nodules detected in pregnancy are likely to be malignant as most of the pregnancy related enlargement is diffuse.

The fetus is dependant on maternal thyroid hormone until autonomous fetal thyroid function begins at 12 weeks. Thyroxine is important for fetal brain development, myelination and Purkinje cell function.

Susclinical Hypothyroidism → ↓ intelligence & neurodevelopmental delay.

Severe Hypothyroidism → brain damage & neurological Cretinism in child

PART 2
Gynecology

PAPER 1

1. **A 20-year-old nulliparous woman complains of severe bloating sensation, difficulty in sleeping and breast tenderness. She appears irritable and reveals that her periods are due in about a week. Enumerate the management options available to her.**

Note: A good way to answer such questions is to add a word on diagnosis and divide the management options into supportive, medical and surgical options.

Premenstrual syndrome (PMS) is the most likely diagnosis if the symptoms have been present for at least 4 out of the previous six months. It has been renamed as premenstrual dysphoric disorder (PMDD). Other disorders manifesting episodically should be excluded by psychiatric evaluation.

PMDD shows a strong placebo effect. She should be handled sympathetically, and the likely etiology explained for reassurance. General measures like exercise, relaxation techniques like meditation and yoga may be beneficial. She should be encouraged to eat a well balanced diet with low salt and fat content to reduce premenstrual bloating. Alcohol, chocolate, dairy products and caffeinated beverages may accentuate her irritability and their intake should be restricted.

Evening primrose oil has been found to be effective especially for relieving the breast symptoms, and is also devoid of side effects. Supplements of vitamin B_6 (pyridoxine), vitamin E, and gamma linoleic acid have also proved to be of some value.

The management options available to her are mainly for symptomatic relief. Since the disorder is often associated with ovulatory cycles only, suppression of ovulation has been tried. Combined contraceptive pills may be effective in some. Danazol 100-200 mg daily is effective in treating breast symptoms but may cause unacceptable side effects like hirsutism. GnRH agonists like Triptorelin or Luprolide are of limited value as they are costly, may cause osteopenia and can only be used for short periods of 6 months.

Severe bloating and weight gain may require the use of diuretics like Spironolactone, which is an aldosterone antagonist or Frusemide for short periods each month. However, its overuse is to be avoided as it can lead to diuretic induced hypokalemia. NSAIDs may be added in the late luteal phase for any associated dysmenorrhea.

Insomnia can be treated with anxiolytics like alprazolam or sedatives. Selective serotonin reuptake inhibitors like Fluoxitene 20 mg are becoming the first line therapy for PMDD because they are effective, well tolerated and free of major side effects. In depressive mood disorders, tricyclic antidepressants have been used.

The use of surgery is not an option due to her young age.

Thus, the management options in PMDD are mainly symptomatic and have to be tailored to suit the patient's symptoms. Its management is important because the symptoms of PMDD can lead to socioeconomic loss, and secondly because of associated legal implications that arise in conjunction with personal accountability in cases of PMDD.

2. **You have just delivered a baby with ambiguous l[...]
   Baby is otherwise normal. What advice will you [...]
   regarding the condition and further manageme[...]**

A newborn with ambiguous genitalia requires imm[...] not only because of parental anxiety but also because one of its c[...] losing congenital adrenal hyperplasia may be rapidly fatal in the first week o[...] life if the electrolyte levels are not closely monitored and corrected.

The parents should be counseled that ambiguous genitalia may be the result of a chromosomal disorder or more commonly may occur in a chromosomally normal infant, due to endocrinal abnormalities.

History of drug intake during pregnancy of androgenic progesterones should be elicited. Child should be examined to identify palpable gonads. In the absence of palpable gonads, it is most likely that the child is female and the parents should be informed as such.

Karyotyping should be done by examining the buccal smear for Barr bodies, doing a skin biopsy or analyzing the neutrophils in cord blood. Sex chromosome abnormalities that may be encountered are True hermaphroditism, i.e. XO/XY (rare), Turner's syndrome mosaics, Klinefelter's syndrome, normal XX or XY constitution.

17α-hydroxyprogesterone levels should be measured in blood and are elevated in CAH. Normal testosterone levels may indicate testicular feminization syndrome due to end organ insensitivity.

Serum electrolytes should be checked urgently to rule out the possibility of salt losing type of CAH. In this case sodium and chloride may be low and potassium raised. The salt losing type has in addition low aldosterone levels and requires immediate replacement steroid therapy. Electrolyte imbalance should be promptly corrected. If the electrolytes are normal, parents should be reassured that the child is healthy but there is a developmental anomaly of the genitalia.

Pelvic ultrasound should be performed to discover the presence of a uterus and vagina. Associated renal tract abnormalities should be looked for which can be found in 20% of patients. Laparotomy and gonadal biopsy may be required to establish the diagnosis in hermaphrodites.

Multidisciplinary team should be involved in the neonates care. Prompt correction of electrolyte imbalance, and cortisol for adrenocorticotropic hormone suppression are areas of immediate concern. Surgical correction of the external genitalia should be undertaken once the disorder has been brought under control.

Note: *The first diagnosis to be confirmed or refuted for such an infant is CAH. It is the commonest cause of a masculinised female and is due to deficiency of 21-hydroxylase enzyme which converts 17α-hydroxyprogesterone to desoxycortisol and progesterone to desoxycorticosterone.*

3. **A 36-year-old barrister has conceived in an IVF cycle. She is currently 7 weeks pregnant and an ultrasound reveals a gestational sac in right fallopian tube. Debate the various management options available to her.**

When IVF is performed for diseased tubes, even though the embryos are replaced in the uterine cavity, under ultrasound guidance, there is documented retrograde migration of the embryos that can result in an ectopic gestation. This fact has to be explained to the patient sympathetically. An ectopic gestation post IVF is emotionally a traumatic event and patient counseling is required prior to deciding the mode of treatment.

For an unruptured 7 weeks ectopic pregnancy both medical and surgical management options are available. Expectant management is not an option as the incidence of rupture and hemorrhage are high.

- **Medical management** as preferred line of therapy if the criteria are fulfilled such as sac diameter not more than 2.5 cm, no cardiac activity in fetal pole, β hCG levels less than 1500 miu/ml, no signs of fluid in the pelvis by ultrasound. Adequate counseling is required to impress upon the patient the need for strict follow-up, and the possibility of surgical intervention if there are signs of hemorrhage or pain. The drug of choice is methotrexate which is administered in a dose of 50 mg/m^2, with monitoring of β hCG levels and ultrasonography post-therapy to evaluate response. Strict vigilance for signs of rupture of the ectopic pregnancy.

- **Surgical management** is preferably by the laparoscopic route, if the expertise exists. This allows excision of the ectopic gestational sac following linear salpingotomy or even total salpingectomy if the tube is diseased. The contralateral tube should be inspected and if diseased or shows the presence of hydrosalpinx, its corneal end should be coagulated or clipped to prevent the occurrence of an ectopic on the other side. Laparoscopy allows faster postoperative recovery and can be performed as a day case, hence is cost effective. This is the procedure of choice if the criteria for medical management are not fulfilled.

- Laparotomy and linear salpingotomy or total salpingectomy is also an option, but requires longer postoperative recovery and hospital stay.

- SAM (Surgically administered medical therapy) using KCL injection in the fetal heart or methotrexate in the gestational sac under ultrasound guidance using an ovum pick up needle is also an option. It has the advantage of being less invasive, but requires strict follow-up with beta hCG and may require surgical intervention in the rare event of hemorrhage or rupture. Besides laparoscopy gives us the chance of inspecting the contralateral tube as well.

She should be reassured that a future pregnancy is possible through IVF subsequently.

4. **A 53-year-old postmenopausal school teacher has been suffering from urinary incontinence for the last 5 years. Discuss relevant investigations and treatment options.**

Complete gynecological and medical, surgical history should be elicited, including a history of chronic cough, smoking, constipation or uterocervical descent. These, if present, will need simultaneous correction. Past history of any medical therapy for incontinence followed by general, systemic and gynecological examination to demonstrate stress urinary incontinence if present.

Bonney's 3 swab test will distinguish stress incontinence from vesico-vaginal fistula, and a Q tip placed at the bladder neck will tell us about bladder neck descent. Investigations in the form of urine routine and microscopic examination should be done to check the specific gravity of the urine which is low in diabetes insipidus or inappropriate ADH syndrome. Urine culture and sensitivity should be done to rule out urinary tract infection, which should be treated prior to any surgical intervention. Ultrasound of the lower abdomen will pick up any ureteric or vesical stones that can result in both urinary infection as well as urinary urgency. A post void volume check should be made on ultrasound scan which will tell us about overflow incontinence.

Urodynamic testing to know if detrusor instability is present, offer and blood sugar for diabetes. Maintenence of a fluid intake/void diary will tell us about the social incapacitation from incontinence and also if fluid restriction would help.

Treatment options would depend on the type of incontinence.

Medical management is the first line treatment in cases of detrusor instability. It consists of administration of parasympatholytics like oxybutanin or duoloxetine. Duoloxetine causes less dryness of mouth but is more expensive. These drugs are administered once a day and can be the only mode of treatment in pure detrusor overactivity. However, most patients have either a mixed picture or genuine stress incontinence. For these patients we need to supplement bladder drill, Kegel's exercises, use of weighted vaginal cones, vaginal estrogen administration for urogenital atrophy, prior to surgical correction.

Options for surgical management consist of both abdominal and vaginal procedures. Burch colposuspension is the procedure of choice in genuine stress incontinence. It is performed by a suprapubic incision by entering the cave of Retzius extraperitoneally and applying non-absorbable sutures between the vaginal vault and the ileopectineal ligament. It gives an immediate cure rate of 90% with a five-year cure rate of around 70%.

Trans-vaginal Tape (TVT) and Trans-obturator Tape (TOT) are recently introduced procedures that employ non-absorbable proline mesh for lifting the urethra-vesical junction. They have the advantage of being less invasive, require shorter anaesthesia and can be performed as day cases. In comparative studies they give an 80-85% cure rate but long-term cure rate studies are still awaited.

Repair of cystocele and buttressing of bladder neck is not the procedure of choice when genuine stress incontinence is present as both the primary cure rate and the long-term cure rates are inferior to Burch colposuspension.

Other less frequently performed surgical procedures are Pereyra's needle suspension, Marshall Marketi Krantz (which can cause osteitis pubis) and other sling procedures. Collagen injections around the urethral meatus can be done if there is a short and patulous urethral opening. Insertion of an artificial sphincter can be done in cases of failure of primary Burch colposuspension.

PAPER 2

1. **Describe how you would manage a multiparous 22-year-old complaining of break through bleeding whilst taking the combined pill for oral contraception.**

The management of patients with abnormal bleeding involves determining: (a) when the bleeding occurs with respect to the estrogen and progestogen phases of cycle (b) how long the bleeding lasts and how heavy it is (c) is there a possibility of pregnancy related complications (d) is there anything to suggest poor compliance (e) whether or not there has been concomitent drug therapy.

History must be elicited regarding the type and dose of pills that she is taking along with compliance. It should be stressed that she needs to take them at a specific time of the day, every day to minimise hormonel fluctuations which can cause break through bleeding. Intake of exogenous hormones, antibiotics causing antitubercular treatment (Rifampicin) intake of warfarin antiepileptics, inflammatory bowel disorders, malabsorption syndromes, postsurgical stress all can reduce absorption of hormones. Dietary history and family history of endometrial cancers, a coagulation defects should be elicited.

A through per speculum and per vaginal examination should be done to look for cervicites, polyps, enlarged uterus suggestive of fibroids and any adnexal fulness. Transvaginal ultrasound will detect endometrial polyps, fibroids and hyperplasia. Vaginal swabs should be taken in suspected cases of infection. A pipelle or vabra aspiration should be offered for suspicious endometrium. Cervical cytology/PAP smear should be taken if due. A pregnancy test should be offered if there is any suspicion on account of missed pills or decreased dry availability.

Patient should be counseled regarding the problem and management should be directed towards the cause.

If no significant pathology is identified and competence is assured the first step in management would be to increase the daily dose of estrogen such that the endometrium is stabilized followed by administration of progestogen to allow a controlled withdrawal bleed. In the next cycle consider using combined pills with higher estrogen content if patient earlier was on an ultra-low dose preparation. If patient wishes to change her choice of contraception, appropriate counseling in this regard about available options and the advantages and disadvantages of usage should be done.

2. A couple has been living together for 2 years and has been unable to have a baby even after having regular unprotected intercourse. They come to you for advice. Discuss how you would manage them.

A need and risk assessment should be done by eliciting history including life style, sexual obstetrical and contraceptive in a sensitive manner. General physical examination, including height, weight, and BMI should be measured. Presence of galactorrhea should be looked for. Pelvic examination for presence of vaginal discharge, uterine fibroids and adnexal masses should be done.

In the absence of any obvious problem, provide reassurance as spontaneous conception rates are 90-95% within 3 years of unprotected intercourse (for women <35 years) and initiate basic investigations. The couple's assessment of perceived problem should be taken into account and they should be allowed to make an informed decision regarding their management.

Changes in lifestyle should be advised which include; regular sexual intercourse every 2-3 days, limiting alcohol intake to ≤ 1-2 unit's alcohol/week for women; ≤ 3-4/week for men, and maintaining the BMI of both partners between 19-29. Men should avoid tight fitting under clothing for prolonged period of time.

They should be advised to avoid both active and passive smoking. Referral to a smoking cessation program may be offered. Use of recreational drugs and other medications should be enquired. Marijuana is a major cause of decreased sperm count.

Appropriate Folic acid supplementation should be prescribed for at least 3 months. Rubella status should be checked and if susceptible rubella vaccination offered. Avoid pregnancy for one month after vaccination. Cervical screening should be offered.

Initial investigations like semen analysis for the male partner, assessment of ovulation and tubal patency for the female partner should be advised. Screening for cervical chlamydial infection should be offered as treatment of the same can decrease the incidence of pelvic infection and related infertility.

Tests for ovulation assessment include day 21 or mid luteal serum progesterone and follicular study by transvaginal sonography. If anovulatory then serum prolactin, thyroid function and pituitary gonadotropins should be checked. In the absence of known pelvic pathology hyterosalpingogram (HSG) remains the investigation of choice for judging the tubal patency if semen analysis and ovulation tests are normal.

Women with known predisposing factors for infertility should be referred to specialist centers and offered extended counseling. Information leaflets should be provided and if required help with contact numbers of support group agencies may be provided.

Note: All couples with inability to conceive after 2 years of regular unprotected intercourse should be offered investigations. They can be initiated even after one year if age of the female partner is ≥ 35 years or they have an identifiable cause.

Cause of infertility is – unidentified in 30% couples.
Ovulatory disorders in 27%
Tubal damage in 14%
Male factor in 19%
Both male and female factors in 39%

HSG is a reliable indicator of tubal patency but not of occlusion. Hence, it is used as a screening test in couples with no history of pelvic infection and if abnormal, confirmatory laparoscopy should follow. It is also less invasive and cost effective than laparoscopy.

Chlamydial infection can cause both male and female infertility. PCR is currently the test of choice for diagnosis. Confirmed cases require treatment with Doxycycline, partner notification, contact tracing and referral to genitourinary clinics.

3. **A 40-year-old woman having heavy periods for the last 10 years has been found to have a single intramural myoma of 43 mm × 37 mm, on sonography. She comes to you for advice. What are the management options available to her?**

Fibroids are present in 25% of women during reproductive age group.

Menstrual abnormalities like heavy periods, pain, intermenstrual bleeding and pressure symptoms may be associated with fibroids. Presence of any such symptom should be excluded. Fertility requirements of the woman should be known prior to giving her the options. Other causes of heavy bleeding especially those related to intrauterine devices and infection should be ruled out after abdominal, speculum and bimanual examinations. Complete blood count including platelet count, thyroid function tests and coagulation tests should be performed if there is any positive history.

If her heavy cycles are not influencing her general health and lifestyle, and if asymptomatic otherwise, she should be kept under surveillance provided FBC is normal. Appropriate Medical management with Mefanemic acid and Tranexamic acid should be offered for menorrhagia along with hematinics.

If symptomatic menorrhagia or reproductive failure is a problem, Myomectomy may be offered. In cases of intramural myomas with a submucous component, hysteroscopic myomectomy is superior, if expertise exists. Hemorrhage, infection, chance of scar dehiscence during subsequent pregnancy, and recurrence are common complications. It should be offered if she desires to preserve her uterus for future reproduction.

Levonorgestral- releasing intrauterine system (Mirena) is effective in decreasing fibroid related menorrhagia provided the uterine cavity is not distorted. It may cause fibroid shrinkage as well.

GnRH analogues have high incidence of adverse effects and should not be used for more than 6 months. They should be used selectively to reduce fibroid volume and control excessive bleeding preoperatively. Add – back treatment should be considered.

Uterine artery embolisation, laparoscopic myolysis, High intensity focussed ultrasound (HIFU), MRI- guided laser ablation and laser photocoagulation are newer techniques for treatment of symptomatic fibroids in women not desiring further childbirth. Some of these techniques are still undergoing clinical trials.

Hysterectomy provides definitive cure to symptomatic women who have completed their family. It is desirable to perform through the vaginal route with laparoscopic assistance.

4. **Mrs. Jose had a missed miscarriage 4 weeks ago for which a suction evacuation was done. Histopathology suggests a diagnosis consistent with partial hydatidiform mole. How will you explain the diagnosis, its implications for future fertility and further management?**

It is a disorder of the placenta, has a malignant potential but is treatable and requires follow-up. It is often difficult to distinguish with missed miscarriage on ultrasound. Histopathology provides the only definitive diagnosis. Follow-up is required for early identification and treatment of persistent disease and choriocarcinoma.

History of continuing bleeding should be enquired. Registration and Consultation with the screening center at Sheffield, Dundee or Charing Cross should be sought before intervention. Re-evacuation should be considered if she is still bleeding. Even if she is asymptomatic, follow-up, investigations and registration should be advised.

β-HCG in urine should be measured and repeated weekly for 6 weeks till the values reach the limit of detection, then monthly till negative and for another 3 months after that. All the tests are performed at the registration center. Baseline chest X-ray should be performed.

There is a very small risk of persistent trophoblastic disease and only one in 200 women having partial mole require chemotherapy for persistent disease after risk scoring. Hydatidiform mole is usually very sensitive to methotrexate and in majority no other treatment is required. Folinic acid must be administered with methotrexate in all cases.

The minimum follow-up period for partial mole traditionally has been six months but is determined by the regional center. If HCG remains high or rises subsequently, new pregnancy should be excluded and specialist advice sought.

It does not affect her fertility but should be advised not to conceive until the HCG level has been normal for 6 months or one year after completion of chemotherapy. Double barrier protection should be advised. Oral contraceptive pills are safe to use after the HCG levels have returned to normal.

Any subsequent pregnancy should be confirmed by early ultrasound scan to exclude recurrence.

β-HCG should be repeated 6 weeks after all subsequent deliveries. Risk of recurrence is 1 in 55.

Note: The incidence of GTN is 1 in 714 live births in UK. GTN includes hydatidiform mole, invasive mole, choriocarcinoma, and placental site trophoblastic tumor.

Complete H. moles are diploid, with no fetal tissue and androgenetic in origin, i.e. no maternal tissues (consequence of duplication of haploid sperm or rarely a dispermic fertilization of an empty ovum).

Partial moles are triploid (one set of maternal and 2 sets of paternal haploid genes) and have evidence of fetal tissues.

PAPER 3

1. **A 25-year-old woman requests an abortion citing personal reasons. Her LMP was 8 weeks back. Discuss the management options.**

Both medical and surgical methods are safe, effective and acceptable at this gestational age. If the gestational age or location is doubtful a scan should be offered to determine the same.

Testing for hemoglobin concentration, ABO and rhesus blood groups, red cell antibodies, and HIV should be performed. Testing for hemoglobinopathies, vaginal swabs for Chlamydia and hepatitis B, and C should be offered in the presence of high-risk factors.

Adequate counseling should be offered, and information leaflets provided so that she can make an informed decision regarding the options available.

Medical abortion using mifepristone plus prostaglandin is appropriate till 9 weeks gestational age (63 days). Mifepristone 200 mg orally followed 1-3 days later by gemeprost 0.5 mg vaginally is the recommended regimen. The success rate is close to 95% and 1% women continued pregnancy requiring a second trial with medical abortion or proceeding to surgical termination.

It should be avoided in women with suspected ectopic pregnancy, undiagnosed adnexal masses, intrauterine device in place, long-term systemic corticosteroid therapy, chronic adrenal failure, severe anemia and known allergy. Misoprostol should be avoided in women with uncontrolled epilepsy and allergy to prostaglandins.

Suction termination is a safe option. Most of the terminations are done under general anesthesia (GA) but local anesthesia (Para cervical block) is safer than GA and should be offered. Conscious sedation may be offered if expertise exists. Cervical preparation with misoprostol (400 micrograms administered vaginally 3 hours before surgery) or mifepristone tablets (600 mg/ 200 mg orally 48 hours prior to surgery) reduces the complication rate. Risk of uterine perforation (0.4%), hemorrhage (0.1%), cervical trauma, failed abortion necessitating further procedure should be informed. A small risk of hysterectomy must also be mentioned on the consent form.

Electric or manual aspiration with special devices is effective, safe and has shorter operating time.

Anti D immunoglobulin 250 IU should be given to all RhD D negative women within 72 hours following abortion, whether by surgical or medical means.

Note: In UK, abortion is legal till 24 weeks. For first 7 weeks, Medical abortion is the first line method.

Terminations done after 12 weeks require the signature of two registered practitioners on the abortion form.

2. Summarize the management of missed combined oral contraceptive pills.

The chances of failure (pregnancy) depend on the **'Number'** of missed pills and also on **'When'** those pills are missed. The risk of pregnancy is greatest when pills are missed at the beginning or end of the pack containing active hormonal pills. Seven consecutive pills are required to inhibit ovulation and the rest for maintaining anovulation.

If she has missed one or two 30-35 μg or one 20 μg ethinyestradiol (EE) pills, at any time, she should take the most recent missed pill as soon as possible and then continue taking the remaining pills daily, one each day, at her usual time. Additional or emergency contraception is not required.

If 2 and more 20 μg or 3 and more 30-35 μg EE pills have been missed at any time during the cycle, she should take the most recent pill as soon as possible and then continue taking rest of the pills daily. Additional precautions like barriers or abstinence should be taken till she has taken pills for 7 days. If these pills are missed in week 1 (1-7 days of starting the pack), effectively extending the pill free interval and she had unprotected sex (in week 1 or in the PFI), emergency contraception should be considered.

If the missed pills are in weak three (Days 15-21), she should finish the pills in her current pack and start a new pack the next day omitting the pill-free interval (PFI). Emergency contraception is not required if Pill-free interval is avoided.

If she has missed more than seven active consecutive pills, then she must be viewed as having stopped taking the pill and the missed pills rules cannot be applied.

If a woman misses any inactive pills, she should discard the missed inactive pills and then continue taking pills daily, one each day.

Note: COCs inhibit ovulation by reducing gonadotropins. They also make cervical mucus and endometrium hostile for implantation. Seven consecutive pills are regularly missed in the PFI without losing contraceptive protection. Follicular activity occurs without ovulation in the PFI. Risk of failure is higher with combined oral contraceptives (COCs) containing low dose estrogens.

In UK, 21 day pill regimen (without the 7 inactive placebo pills) is commonly followed and advice is given accordingly.

3. **A healthy 75-year-old woman has developed symptomatic vaginal vault prolapse many years after total abdominal hysterectomy for a benign pathology. How would you advise her regarding treatment options?**

Detailed history of the discomfort and associated symptoms should be enquired. Her present sexual history and desire for medical or surgical intervention should be known.

Preoperative urodynamic assessment should be considered especially in the presence of pre-existing urinary complaints. Post-hysterectomy vault prolapse is usually associated with enterocele and other support defects. Recurrent surgery is more complex, risky and prone to failure. She should be allowed to make an informed decision regarding her treatment.

Conservative management includes use of shelf pessaries. HRT and physiotherapy are of no benefit.

McCall's culdoplasty performed vaginally is an effective option. Uterosacral ligaments are identified and fixed to the pubocervical and rectovaginal fascia at the level of ischial spine. There is a one in 10 chance of ureteric damage and procedure is difficult with complete vault evertions.

Sacrospinous fixation performed vaginally has high success rate, short hospital stay and less morbidity. It involves fixing the vagina with Sacrospinous ligament but may cause pudendal nerve damage.

Sacrocolpopexy requires an abdominal approach, longer operating time and hospital stay. There is risk of ureteric and bowel damage but is considered more effective. Laparoscopic approach should be offered if expertise exists.

Intravaginal slingplasty is a new day care procedure wherein a polypropylene tape is secured to vagina and uterosacral ligaments. Long-term effectiveness studies are awaited.

Colpocleisis is an option if she does not require a functional vagina. It may not be very suitable for healthy women. If genuine stress incontinence is identified, colposuspension may also be considered.

4. Enumerate the precautions that you will take to minimize urinary morbidity during hysterectomy?

Divide the precautions between preoperative, intraoperative and post-operative period. Risk assessment is integral part of answering any such question. It is important to identify that the question includes not only TAH but also lap assisted (LAVH) and radical hysterectomy.

Appropriate preoperative assessment and investigations should be performed depending on the underlying pathology and proposed route of operation. Pre- existent urinary dysfunction should be ruled out by history and urodynamic investigations if necessary.

Urine infection is commonly related to catheterization and stasis of urine. Prophylactic antibiotics can reduce the infection rates.

Risk of ureteric injury is higher in previous pelvic and uterine surgeries (LSCS), enlarged uterus, distorted pelvic anatomy, massive intraoperative hemorrhage, and endometriosis. High index of suspicion should be kept in such cases.

Laparoscopic procedures should be undertaken wherever possible, as the risk of injury is lower.

Intravenous urogram (IVU) should be performed to identify anatomical variations and previous ureteric pathology in women with large adnexal masses (4 cm and more), big uterus ($\geq$ 12 weeks) and with abnormal pelvic examination.

Ureteric damage can be reduced by careful dissection, adequate exposure and good surgical technique, use of splints, help of urological colleagues and the judicious use of the subtotal operation.

Bladder should be mobilized in a downward and outward direction so the ureters move away from the operative field. Blind clamping of bleeding vessels should be avoided in the vulnerable areas. Tissue hemostasis should be good so that formation of vault hematoma is avoided.

Bladder damage can be avoided by careful dissection, an empty bladder, use of subtotal procedure, and the use of longer catheterization with difficult dissections or presence of hematuria and the recognition and repair of injuries when they occur.

Short-term voiding disorders are due to pain, immobility and excess iv fluids. Adequate analgesia, hydration and early ambulation should be encouraged.

During laparoscopic surgery, short applications of diathermy should be encouraged to limit the thermal damage to urinary structures.

If any ureteric injury is suspected, intraoperative ureteric catheterization should be done and early urological assistance sought. Prompt and meticulous repair decreases the associated morbidity. Transurethral cystoscopy can visualize ureteric jets from both ureteric orifices. Its routine use should be promoted in complex cases. Use of wound drains should be encouraged.

Seventy percent injuries are identified in the postoperative period. Vigilance should be maintained for symptoms like fever, hematuria, flank pain, abdominal distention, anuria and urinary leakage.

Note: Risk of ureteric damage is 1 in 500 for benign disease, and 1 in 100 for malignancy. Bladder damage occurs in 1 in 200 cases.

PAPER 4

1. **A 37-year-old woman presents at your OPD with slight vaginal bleeding. She has conceived with IVF and embryes were transfered 6 weeks back. Tansvaginal ultrasound shows an intrauterine pregnancy with a 6 mm fetus but no fetal heart pulsations. How will you manage her?**

Fetal heart pulsations should be detectable in a fetus $\geq$ 6 mm or at 6 weeks. Since in an IVF pregnancy the gestational age is certain, these findings suggest a failing pregnancy.

While explaining the diagnosis to her, the term miscarriage should preferably be used instead of "abortion". The couple should be offered sympathetic counseling and provided with information leaflets. Her blood group and Rhesus factor should be checked.

Unless the bleeding becomes heavy, pelvic examination and repeat ultrasound scanning within 1-2 days is not beneficial. Immediate hospital admission is not essential and she should be allowed to make an informed decision. The options include—Expectant management, medical therapy, or surgical evacuation.

Expectant management includes repeating ultrasound scan after 1 week or anytime the bleeding becomes heavy. She may expel products of conception spontaneously. It may reassure the woman of the diagnosis and avoid the need for admission and GA. Serial β HCG levels may be offered to check the rising titers. Bed-rest, progesterone or HCG supplements are not effective.

Medical management with mifepristone and prostaglandin is the preferred option when she is psychologically prepared.

Surgical curettage may be required if expectant management fails or with heavy bleeding. Anti D immunoglobulin should be administered if she is RhD negative, nonsensitised and undergoes evacuation.

Follow-up extended counseling should be offered as a failed IVF pregnancy is a big psychological set back for the woman.

2. A 32-year-old parus woman is complaint of postcoital bleeding. She is anxious as she has heard that it could be a sign of cancer. How will you manage her condition?

Common causes of postcoital bleeding at her age include infection, genital tract trauma, cervical or endometrial polyp, cervical ectropion and coincidental intermenstrual bleeding. Malignancy as a cause of bleeding is unlikely. Pregnancy related complications should be ruled out at the outset.

Detailed history should be elicited regarding the amount, frequency, duration of bleeding and its relation to intercourse. Menstrual history, intake of exogenous hormones, and history of trauma to genital tract are important. Excessive vaginal discharge, foul smell or any recent change in the discharge should be noted. Family history of cancers and the reason for her fear should be asked gently.

Possibility of bleeding disorder should be kept in mind if associated with other menstrual symptoms like intermittent intermenstrual bleeding or if she is on anticoagulant therapy.

General physical examination (anemia) and abdominal examination for abnormal masses should be done.

Vulval **inspection** for signs of trauma, and vulvitis, examination with cuscoes speculum (cervicitis, ectropion, and vaginal discharge) and bimanual examination of pelvis should be offered.

Appropriate **swabs** for microscopy and cervical smear should be taken (if due) prior to bimanual examination. Pregnancy test or serum β HCG if there is any possibility of pregnancy.

Transvaginal ultrasound for pelvic pathology and endometrial assessment for polyps. Endocervical polyps can be avulsed in outpatient setting. If postcoital bleeding continues after that a formal hysteroscopic evaluation of endometrium during proliferative phase should be offered for endometrial sampling.

Appropriate **antimicrobial therapy and contact tracing** should be offered if sexually transmitted diseases are a cause of cervicitis.

Ectropion can cause PCB in 5% women. Superimposed infections are common. **Cryotherapy** is usually enough but occasionally ablative methods are required after treating infection and ensuring a normal smear.

Referral for **colposcopy and cervical biopsy** should be done if there is suspicion of invasion or if the smear is abnormal.

Note: Triple swabs should be taken for ruling out sexually transmitted disease. One high vaginal swab for culture and 2 endocervical swabs for gonorrhoea culture and Chlamydia analysis.

3. **A 42-year-old healthy woman comes to you for contraceptive advice. How will you counsel her?**

She should be informed that although a natural decline in fertility occurs from the age of 37 years, irregular ovulation still occurs and effective contraception is required to prevent unplanned pregnancy.

The contraceptive choice for her may be influenced by many factors—frequency of intercourse, natural decline in fertility, sexual function, the wish for non-contraceptive benefits, menstrual dysfunction and concurrent medical conditions.

A clinical history, including sexual history should be taken to assess the contraceptive options, taking account of cardiovascular and cerebrovascular disease and neoplasia, which increase with age.

No contraceptive is contraindicated by age alone. She should be informed about the risks and non-contraceptive benefits of all contraceptive methods and allowed to make an informed decision.

She can use combined hormonal contraception including the pills (COC) unless there are co-existing diseases or risk factors. It should be avoided if she is a smoker, has cardiovascular disease, migraine, or stroke. There is a slight increase in the risk of venous thromboembolism, ischaemic stroke, breast cancer, cervical intraepithelial neoplasia and cervical cancer with COC use for long time. Monophasic pills with less than 30 μg ethinylestradiol and low dose of norethisterone or levonorgestrel should be preferred as the first line option.

She should be informed that there is an increase in bone mineral density and reduced incidence of hip fractures, a 50% reduction in risk of ovarian, endometrial cancer and colorectal cancer, decreased incidence of benign breast disease, menstrual bleeding, pain and hot flushes with COC use. There may be a reduction in incidence of functional ovarian cysts, benign ovarian tumors, acne and rheumatoid arthritis. No causal association between COC use and weight gain has been found.

There is no apparent increase in risk of cardiovascular disease or stroke with progesterone only contraceptives. LNG-IUS (Mirena) and implants are safe to use even if she had a previous history of ischemic heart disease or VTE. There is no significant increase in breast cancer risk. However, there may be a slight decrease in BMD and irregular bleeding associated with POC use.

Information about permanent methods like vasectomy and tubal occlusion with their advantages, disadvantages and relative failures should be discussed.

She may use barrier methods without spermicidal lubricant, which help to prevent STI's also.

Copper intrauterine devices are safe to use. An endocervical swab to detect *Chlamydia* and gonorrhea should be offered and risk of menstrual abnormalities in the first few months explained. Once inserted, it can be left in situ until the menopause.

Natural family planning methods like withdrawal are not reliable and hence not recommended.

She should continue contraception till post menopause is confirmed (After one year of amenorrhoea) or at 55 years.

Note: Average age of perimenopause in UK is 46 years and lasts for approximately 5 years. Average age of menopause is 50.7 years.

4. An 18-year-old woman complains of painful periods. She is not sexually active. Discuss her management.

She should be explained about the physiological basis of pain sympathetically and provided with information booklets describing menstrual cycle and likely reasons of her symptom.

Specific pathology is unlikely to be present in a young sexually inactive woman and this opportunity should be utilized to speak to the patient in the absence of her mother to explore family and social pressures.

Pelvic examination is rarely helpful, ultrasound scanning is preferred if necessary. It reassures the woman and helps to exclude major pathology.

Pain is related to prostaglandin release due to ovulation therefore non-steroidal anti-inflammatory drugs started on the first day of period or pain, whichever is earlier, are the logical first line therapy. Combined oral contraceptives are also an effective treatment which may have additional benefits like reducing the flow and fulfilling the need for future contraception. Other options like luteal phase progestogens, Danazol, calcium channel blockers and medicated IUCD may not be suitable for her but a trial of treatment for three months may be advisable after explaining the risks and benefits.

If vomiting is present, non-oral treatment with anti-emetics may be required.

Laparoscopy, to diagnose and treat underlying pathology, (endometriosis) is indicated only in resistant cases.

Note: During dysmenorrhea plasma concentrations of vasopressin, and myometrial concentrations of PGF 2α are high. While uterine blood flow decreases during pain.

PAPER 5

1. **A 49-year-old woman with heavy periods has an endometrial biopsy as part of investigations. Histopathology shows endometrial hyperplasia. Justify her further investigations and management.**

The type of hyperplasia must be ascertained as the malignant potential and further treatment is dependent on that. Both exogenous (drugs- tamoxifen) and endogenous (ovarian tumour) sources of estrogens should be excluded on history, examination and ultrasound scan.

Simple/cystic hyperplasia has very low malignant potential, hence conservative management is appropriate. Treatment with tranexamic acid and/ or mefenemic acid or long-term progesterone should be prescribed for symptom control.

Adenomatous/complex hyperplasia has a limited malignant potential. Hysterectomy should be offered as it will identify other endometrial pathology and allow further endometrial sampling. On opting conservative management, six months to yearly follow-up with 3/12 progestogens or Mirena intrauterine device and repeat hysteroscopic guided endometrial sampling should be offered.

Atypical hyperplasia has a very high chance of subsequent development of cancer or coexisting with endometrial cancer. Thus hysterectomy and bilateral salpingo-oophorectomy should be offered as the treatment of choice.

Note: The progress to endometrial cancer is less than one in hundred with cystic hyperplasia, 3-4 in a hundred with Adenomatous hyperplasia and 22-33 in hundred with atypical hyperplasia. In 25-50% cases, atypical hyperplasia is coexistent with carcinomatous change in the uterus.

2. **A couple approaches you for tubal ligation as they have completed their family. Outline the briefs of your counseling.**

The couple should be put at ease and the reason for their request should be explored. She should not seek sterilization as a cure for menstrual or sexual dysfunction. Appropriate medical history, any problems with past or current contraception, and their sex life should be discussed. Possibility of desiring more children, breakdown of marriage or situation arising due to death of a child should be gently enquired.

They should be informed that the procedure is intended to be permanent with 30-80% chances of success of reversal operation, should that be necessary. NHS rarely pays for the cost of reversal operations or further fertility procedures like IVF or ICSI.

They should be informed about other long-term reversible methods of contraception like- LNG-IUS, subdermal implants, and copper intrauterine contraceptives, along with their advantages, disadvantages and relative failure rates.

Both vasectomy and tubal occlusion should be discussed. Tubal occlusion carries a lifetime failure risk of one in 200 while vasectomy carries a lower failure rate in terms of post procedure pregnancy to one in 2000 and there is less risk related to the procedure. In case of failure of tubal ligation, the resulting pregnancy may be ectopic and she must seek medical advice if she misses her periods or has abnormal abdominal pain or vaginal bleeding.

Information leaflets/other recorded information should be provided which they may take away and read before the operation to enable them to make an informed decision. Additional counseling sessions may be arranged for young couples or women with special needs, to decrease the incidence of regret later.

If the woman is obese, or has had previous abdominal surgery, she should be informed about the risks of laparoscopy and the chances of requiring laparotomy if there are problems with laparoscopy. Method of access and tubal occlusion to be used in her case should be explained to her. General anesthesia is usually required for laparoscopic tubal ligation and is a day case procedure. It is not associated with heavier or abnormal bleeding subsequently but few women may experience abdominal pain and psychosexual morbidity.

It is commonly performed in the early follicular period and effective contraception should be prescribed till that time.

Note: Oral contraceptives are the commonest type of contraception used in UK followed by condoms. Method failure rates per 100 women years of use for common contraceptives are:

Combined pill, LNG-IUS	–	0.1
Copper IUD	–	0.7
Tubal sterilization	–	0.13
Vasectomy	–	0.01
Male and female condoms	–	4-8
Emergency contraception	–	20-25% failure rate

3. Enumerate the precautions that you will ensure for safe laparoscopic entry into the abdomen.

Adequately trained and experienced operator, well maintained equipment and theater staff is known to decrease overall complication rates during laparoscopy. Each patient should be analyzed to identify her risk of bowel adhesion. Palmer's point on left hypogastrium should be utilized, after excluding splenomegaly to visualize the periumbilical area in women at high risk for bowel adhesions.

Preoperatively bladder should be emptied and abdomen palpated for surface landmarks and abnormal masses. Position of umbilicus may be variable and iliac crests should instead be used to mark the level of aortic bifurcation.

In lean women entry in Trendelenburg position should be avoided. Some surgeons recommend horizontal position for all women. Veress needle should be checked for sharpness, spring action and patency, to allow free flow of gas.

The umbilicus should be elevated mechanically during insertion of Veress to increase the distance of abdominal wall to great vessels. Further insertion should stop once peritoneal cavity is entered. Do not swing the Veress needle under the peritoneum. Tests (saline aspiration, gas flow-pressure readings) to confirm the intraperitoneal position of Veress should be performed.

For adequate distension of abdominal cavity CO_2 should be insufflated to 25 mmHg until all trocars are inserted and lowered to 12-15 mmHg only after insertion. The primary trocar should be inserted through the base of the umbilicus and a $360°$ survey should be performed to exclude bowel or vascular trauma. Direct trocar entry should be avoided in women at high risk of adhesions.

The inferior and superior epigastric vessels should be identified prior to insertion of secondary trocars in lower abdomen.

Note: *The incidence of major bowel injury during laparoscopic entry is 1 in 2500 and that of major vascular injury is 1 in 5000.*

4. **A 32-year-old woman was found to have bilateral chocolate cysts on diagnostic laparoscopy. She has been trying to conceive for the past 4 years. Discuss the relevant issues.**

This question can be dealt under male, female and general issues.

Endometriosis may be the reason for her infertility. The choice of treatment depends upon several factors including previous treatment, the nature and severity of symptoms, size of cysts, and grade of endometriosis. She should be asked to prioritize her concerns between pain and infertility and treatment initiated accordingly. If infertility is the prime concern, investigations should be commenced for the same.

Tubal patency, sperm count and ovulation need to be checked. She should be advised for smoking cessation, cervical screening if due, Rubella status and preconception folic acid supplementation.

Non-steroidal anti-inflammatory drugs may help in reducing the pain associated with endometriosis. There is no role for medical therapy with hormonal drugs in the treatment of endometriosis infertility. Laparoscopic ablation of all the disease deposits results in higher pregnancy rates. Laparoscopic drainage of the cysts followed by stripping or fulgeration of the cyst lining is the procedure of choice. It conserves enough ovarian tissue even when the cysts are large. Simultaneous ablation of all disease deposits result in higher pregnancy rates. If necessary, the ureters should be catheterized prior to surgery. If extensive bowel or bladder adhesions are encountered, laparotomy may become necessary.

The use of GnRh agonists prior to or after surgery needs to be individualized. If the cysts are large and leave no room for safe insertion of the laparoscope, preoperative depot GnRh agonists can be employed for three months to shrink the cysts. Postoperatively one should proceed to ovulation induction in the every next cycle and use of medical therapy is to be discouraged.

Need for assisted conception depends on her findings. If required super ovulation with GnRH analogues and IUI offer better prognosis. If she has severe endometriosis, refer her to a specialist center for further treatment. All efforts should be made to put her in touch with support groups.

Note: The American Fertility Society's scoring system to classify endometriosis is:

Peritoneum			
Endometrial deposits	< 1 cm	1-3 cm	>3 cm
Score	1	2	3
Adhesions	Filmy	Dense with partial obliteration of Pouch of Douglas	Dense with complete obliteration of pouch
Score	1	2	3
Ovary			
Endometrial deposits	< 1 cm	1-3 cm	>3 cm
Right score	2	4	6
Left score	2	4	6
Adhesions	Filmy	Dense with partial Enclosure of ovary	Dense with complete enclosure of ovary
Right score	2	4	6
Left score	2	4	6
Tube			
Endometriosis	<1 cm	>1 cm	Tube occluded
Right score	2	4	6
Left score	2	4	6
Adhesions	Filmy	Dense with tube distorted	Dense with tube occluded
Right score	2	4	6
Left score	2	4	6

Stage I–mild 1-5
Stage II–moderate 6-15
Stage III–severe 16-30
Stage IV–extensive 31-54

PAPER 6

1. Discuss the issues involved in taking consent for an abdominal hysterectomy for a benign cause in a 45-year-old woman?

Note: *In any consent question, the issues can be divided into general issues for any surgery and specific issues pertaining to that particular situation. Due to her age, discussion about removal or retention of ovaries should be the highlight of the essay.*

The patient should be made aware of the name and nature of operation and the reason for it being performed. She should be aware that it involves removing her uterus and cervix through an abdominal incision. This will stop her menstruation and other symptoms not related to uterus will not be affected.

Other medical, less invasive procedures (LNG-IUS, endometrial ablation) and alternative therapies should have already been discussed along with the option of no treatment prior to surgery. Information leaflets/ tapes should be provided and woman allowed to take an informed decision. Details of counseling and her wishes regarding treatment must be documented in her file.

She should be informed of the serious and frequently occurring risks of the procedure. If she is obese, has had previous surgery or pre-existing medical conditions, her risks of complications are higher. She should be warned about the presence of TED stockings, intracaths, urinary catheter and a possible enema in the postoperative period.

Risks of damage to bladder/ureters/bowel and bladder dysfunction should be explained and repair of the same may be required during the procedure. One in a 100 women require blood transfusion due to haemorrhage and consent for the same should be taken beforehand specially in Jehovah's witness. There is a small risk of pelvic abscess/ infection, VTE, and return to theatre for additional stitches. All operations carry a risk of dying 1 in 4000. The frequent side effects include – wound infection, bruising, frequency of micturition, delayed wound healing, keloid formation and early menopause.

Oophorectomy without consent may constitute assault. She should be clearly informed of the risk and benefits of removing her ovaries. Conditions where oophorectomy is beneficial are a positive family history of breast or ovarian cancers, abnormal looking ovaries per operatively, or there is uncontrolled bleeding from the site and oophorectomy can control this bleeding. Some benign diseases may be better treated by including oophorectomy, e.g. endometriosis, PID, unexpected pathology found at surgery and where there are unwanted ovarian endocrine effects, e.g. PMS, hirsutism, mastalgia.

The advantages of oophorectomy relate to the prevention of ovarian cancer and avoidance of a possible future surgery for subsequently developing ovarian pathology.

The disadvantages of oophorectomy relate to the loss of libido, which may be difficult or impossible to treat and the longer the use of HRT the greater the increased risk of breast cancer – although this risk may be less with the use of SERMs.

She should be made aware of the form of anesthesia planned and discuss it with anaesthetist prior to surgery.

2. **A 38-year-old parous woman has been experiencing dull ache in her lower abdomen for many months with occasional exacerbations. All preliminary investigations have been unremarkable. How will you further manage her condition?**

Any management question can be divided into history, examination, investigations and treatment. Treatment should be divided into empirical and specific strategies.

Possibility of non-gynecological problems like functional and inflammatory bowel conditions (Irritable bowel syndrome, Crohn's disease or ulcerative colitis), along with pelvic inflammatory disease, endometriosis, adnexal neoplasm and pelvic congestion syndrome should be considered.

History should be detailed and include relationship to periods, pain with coitus, exacerbating factors, dietary history, sexual history, drug history (codeine), direct questions on gastrointestinal systems, diet and past psychological problems and abuse.

Examination includes general physical and bimanual vaginal examination. These may reveal pelvic masses, cervical fullness and fixed retroversion. Endocervical swabs should be taken for microbiology to exclude Chlamydia or other infections.

Investigations should be directed by the history. Midstream urinalysis, X-ray KUB, and bowel studies may be necessary. Pelvic ultrasound is of limited value but may be reassuring to the woman and occasionally reveal pathology not noted on clinical examination.

Laparoscopy may be required if no other cause is identifiable but it carries risk and may lead to confounding diagnosis and erroneous treatment. (e.g. minimal endometriosis).

Empirical treatment includes dietary changes, alternative therapies like homeopathic remedies. Specific treatment should be directed towards the cause.

3. **You are SpR$_3$ and while performing abdominal hysterectomy for endometriosis, a 3 cm long cut was seen on the bladder. Enumerate the further course of action.**

There are two options for further course. One is to finish the hysterectomy and then pay attention to bladder injury. This utilizes the time spent waiting for other colleagues. Second is to pack the area and tackle the injury first and then complete the hysterectomy.

Inform and call the gynecological consultant for help. Summon urological colleagues.

Visualize the anatomy and trace the ureters and ureteric openings. Complete the procedure in the mean time. Bladder should be closed in two overlapping layers with vicryl 3-0. A pelvic drain should be left in situ. Routine abdominal closure should be as routinely followed. She will require Foley's catheter in situ for 7-10 days.

Postoperative antibiotics and Thromboprophylaxis should be added according to her risk assessment. There is no real need for imaging unless there are concerns.

Debrief the complication to the patient as soon as she is comfortable, acknowledging that the likelihood of such an incident happening is higher due to endometriosis. Appropriate risk management forms should be filled and case notes meticulously completed.

4. **A 35-year-old woman wishes to conceive and TVS done as part of investigations shows a cyst in the right ovary 5 cm and 4 cm in dimensions. Her pregnancy test is negative. Outline her management options.**

Majority of ovarian cysts in reproductive age group are functional and thus benign. None the less, every effort should be made to rule out malignancy. Detailed history should be elicited to exclude symptoms pertaining to other systems.

Detailed ultrasound appearance of the cyst should be sought. Increasing size, presence of septations, papillary formations, echogenic solid areas and free fluid in the pouch of Douglas may suggest ovarian malignancy. Risk of malignancy index (RMI) should be calculated combining her ultrasound findings, CA125 values and premenopausal status.

If her RMI is less than 250, the risk of malignancy is considered low and she may be offered expectant management with a repeat scan 3-6 months later. Approximately 50% simple cysts resolve spontaneously.

If the RMI is more than 250, further management should be planned with a gynaecological oncologist.

In the absence of pain, hormonal suppression with combined oral contraceptives has no role. Cyst aspiration has high chances of recurrence.

Laparoscopic cyst removal may be offered as it carries a lower risk of postoperative adhesion formation that may compromise her future fertility, decreased blood loss, shorter hospital stay, more cosmetic results and lesser morbidity. She should be informed about the risk of laparoscopy, particularly bowel and major vessel injury and that she may require laparotomy should any problems arise.

Laparoscopic cystotomy and ablation or stripping of cyst wall may be offered for treatment of ovarian endometrioma. Bleeding, adhesion formation and loss of adjacent follicles are possible complications.

Cystectomy (removal of intact cyst) may be offered for dermoid cyst and if there is a possible chance of malignancy.

Laparotomy may be required if there is a suspicion of malignancy or if she is unfit for laparoscopy because of obesity or extensive abdominal scarring.

Routine investigations like husband semen analysis, tubal patency, Day 21 serum progesterone and other routine investigations along with vaginal swabs should be checked as part of initial work-up for infertility.

Note: The risk of malignancy index (RMI) is calculated by 3 factors and scores are given for each of them:

RMI= U× M× CA125

U = 0 (for ultrasound score of zero)

U = 1 (for ultrasound score of 1)

U = 3 (for ultrasound score of 2-5)

Ultrasound scans are scored one point for each of the following characteristics: Multilocular cyst, evidence of solid areas, evidence of metastasis, presence of ascitis, bilateral lesions.

M=1 for premenopausal and 3 for all postmenopausal women.

CA125 is the serum CA125 measurement in u/ml.

PAPER 7

1. **A 26-year-old woman had secondary amenorrhoea for six months. During investigations her FSH was 52 IU/l and LH was 34 IU/l. Pregnancy test is negative and all other investigations are unremarkable. She wishes to conceive in the near future. What advice will you give regarding the diagnosis, etiology, investigations and treatment options?**

The investigations point towards a diagnosis of premature ovarian failure (POF). In this condition there is a premature loss of ovarian function; usually before 40 years, either through an accelerated loss or dysfunction of eggs. The reason could vary from a chromosomal or enzymatic defect to viral infection and autoimmune diseases. Sometimes it may not be possible to pinpoint a cause. It should be emphasized that stress is not a cause of POF and she is not responsible for it. It may be hereditary in 5% women.

Menstrual history and other symptoms of menopause like hot flushes, night sweats, sleeping problems, vaginal dryness, and low energy drive or bladder control problems should be enquired. Hormonal analysis should be repeated after 4-6 weeks to confirm the diagnosis and estimate the ovarian reserve. History of any other illness, chemotherapy, recent weight loss or surgery should be elicited.

She should be advised to conceive early. Only 6-8 out of a hundred women with POF will be able to conceive. Semen analysis of her partner and tubal patency should be checked. The couple should be advised to have regular intercourse very 2-3 days.

Lipid profile and bone densitometry should be advised. Ovarian biopsy and karyotyping are not indicated. She should be encouraged to eat a healthy diet and exercise regularly (aerobics and weight training) to decrease health risks of osteoporosis and heart disease. Advise her to quit smoking, as it accelerates ovarian loss. Hormone replacement therapy should be started as the benefits of estrogen replacement outweigh the risks at her age and especially if she is experiencing symptoms.

There is no way to restore follicular function in POF. Ovulation induction should be avoided as already the ovarian reserve is poor.

Oocyte donation, surrogacy and adoption are other options. She should be given opportunities for bereavement counseling and put in touch with support groups.

Note: *Elevated FSH values above 40 iu/l repeated twice over 4-6 weeks suggest POF in a woman less than 40 years. The value fluctuate with time and higher the FSH levels, lower is the ovarian reserve and lower are a woman's chances to conceive. HRT with estrogens will decrease FSH values but will not increase the follicular reserve or function.*

2. **Discuss the management of stage 1b vulval cancer in a 70-year-old diabetic woman.**

Vulval cancer stage 1b is confined to the vulva and the lesion is less than 2 cm in size. There are no lymph nodes involved. Squamous cell tumors predominate. There is a strong relationship with human papilloma virus.

Radical vulvectomy was the treatment of choice in these patients. It involved removal of the entire vulva including both labia majora and minora along with dissection of inguinal lymph nodes. This gives good survival rate but is associated with considerable morbidity and mortality. Besides it compromises sexual function and lowers self-esteem.

Stress urinary incontinence and vaginal wall prolapse can be prevented by use of appropriate repair procedures at the time of surgery. Persistent lymphedema of the legs can be prevented by elevating the legs.

These days a more conservative approach is adopted. Vulvar conservation is advocated for unifocal lesions and groin dissection is done by separate incisions. If two or more lymph nodes are positive, postoperative radiation will reduce the risk of recurrence.

Chemotherapy has no role in squamous cell carcinoma. Vaccination is being developed against human papilloma virus which may be helpful in preventing cervical and vulvar carcinomas.

3. **A 37-year-old woman posted for diagnostic laparoscopy had accidental bowel injury during insertion. Describe the further course of action.**

Inform the consultant gynecologist on call and ask one of the theatre staff also to contact a senior general surgeon to request their assistance and advice. Inform the anaesthetist about the complication and request him to insert a nasogastric tube and commence intravenous antibiotics, e.g. Augmentin/Metronidazole and Cefuroxime.

Remove the ports and open the abdominal cavity by midline incision and define the extent of injury by careful inspection. Prevent spread of faeces throughout the peritoneal cavity by local packing.

Suture the defect with two layers of absorbable suture material with inversion of the colonic mucosa. Consider a functioning colostomy and a corrugated drain, as this perforated bowel had not been prepared.

The wound should be sutured with non-absorbable suture material to the sheath, and the skin should perhaps be sutured with interrupted nylon or prolene sutures because of the risk of wound infection.

Postoperatively continue intravenous fluids and keep nasograstric tube in situ. Broad spectrum antibiotics and adequate Thromboprophylaxis should be administered. Debrief the patient as soon as comfortable explaining the situation and why the colostomy was needed to enable successful bowel healing and that the colostomy will be closed in six weeks time. Documentation should be completed and risk assessment forms filled.

4. **A young college student has had unprotected intercourse during a Saturday night party. She comes to you on Monday morning requesting postcoital contraception to avoid getting pregnant. What advise will you give her?**

Accurate menstrual and sexual history should be elicited to assess her risk of pregnancy but there is no time in the menstrual cycle when there is zero risk of pregnancy following unprotected intercourse (UPSI). In addition to the risk of conception there may be a risk of sexually transmitted infection if the partner's background is not known. She should be given verbal and written information regarding the failure rates of oral and intrauterine emergency contraception (EC) and allowed to make an informed decision.

She should be offered a single dose of levonorgestral 1.5 mg as soon as possible and within 72 hours of UPSI. This offers a success rate of eighty four out of 100. In case she misses the 72 hour deadline, she may take it anytime till 120 hours after UPSI for reducing the pregnancy chances (success rate 60%). If she vomits within 2 hours of taking LNG, she should return as soon as possible for a repeat dose.

Oral mifepristone in a single dose has been found to be effective but is not yet licensed for EC use.

The insertion of an appropriate copper bearing IUCD, up to 5 days after the first episode of UPSI, is the most effective option with an expected success rate of nearly 100%. It can either be removed after the next period or left in situ as a longer term method of contraception. Risk of sexually transmitted infections, young age and nulliparity are not contraindications to IUD use. Chlamydia screening should be offered and prophylactic antibiotics considered prior to insertion of IUCD. Follow-up visits should be arranged to exclude infection, perforation or expulsion.

She may experience bleeding disturbances in her cycle after taking LNG and over half of all women have their periods coming before or after the expected time. Risk of ectopic pregnancy is small but she must report to the hospital for any cycle irregularity and delay. She should use effective contraception or abstinence for the rest of the cycle.

Advice on future contraception and follow-up to exclude pregnancy is essential. Information leaflets for the same should be provided.

Note: LNG EC is effective primarily by inhibiting ovulation. If given prior to LH surge, it inhibits ovulation for 5-7 days. It will not effect existing pregnancy and till now is not known to have any adverse effects on fetus.

PAPER 8

1. **An 18-year-old woman with a BMI of 34 has been found to have a picture consistent with polycystic ovaries on sonar done as a part of investigations for irregular periods. How will you counsel her regarding the diagnosis, treatment and long-term consequenses.**

One in four women have ultrasound appearance of polycystic ovaries. History of hyperandrogenic symptoms like acne, hirsutism etc. should be enquired. Hormonal analysis like FSH, LH, testosterone, DHEA should be done to detect abnormality.

Polycystic ovarian syndrome is diagnosed when 2 out of 3 criteria are fulfilled:

Presence of oligo- and/or anovulation, hyperandrogenism, and ultrasound evidence of polycystic ovaries. Reassure her that PCO is a hormonal disorder and does not normally lead to surgery for the cysts.

The correction of obesity by diet and exercise offers the best chance of minimizing the sequelae of PCO. Persistent obesity carries a risk of gestational and maturity onset diabetes and coronary artery disease. It may be more difficult for her to reduce weight and tab metformin may be tried to improve insulin resistance. Inositol products are also gaining popularity for the same.

Obesity, hirsutism and acne may lead to poor self-image and psychosocial difficulties.

Fasting blood glucose, cholesterol, lipids and trigycerides along with endometrial thickness on ultrasound should be measured.

She needs to use contraception if pregnancy is not desired (especially the COCP, e.g. Dianette). She should have withdrawl bleed with progestogens at least once every 3 months to avoid endometrial hyperplasia.

Long-term consequences are an increased risk of developing type II diabetes mellitus, gestational diabetes, Dyslipidemia, and Cardiovascular disease. Endometrial hyperplasia and later carcinoma is a possibility especially if she does not have regular bleeds, but discussion of these are probably inappropriate at this age. She should be advised to have annual fasting blood glucose and urinalysis for glycosuria which if abnormal should be followed by a glucose tolerance test.

Note: Polycystic ovary has been defined as an ovary with 12 or more follicles measuring 2-9 mm in diameter and/or increased ovarian volume (≥ 10 cm^3) on ultrasound.

2. A 28-year-old woman complains of recurrent urinary infections for which she has to see the doctor frequently. She is not pregnant and wishes to know the reason why she is suffering. Outline your management.

A detailed history of urinary complaints, frequency and duration of illness, any precipitating factor like menstruation or sexual activity should be noted. History of diabetes or SLE in self or family should be enquired. Tuberculosis should be kept in mind if she is of Asian origin or has a history of travel to these areas. Previous records should be checked to note the abnormality in urinary examination.

A general physical examination and abdominal examination to look for anemia and enlarged lymph nodes should be made. A pelvic examination should exclude a pelvic mass, large urinary residue and cystocoel.

A clean catch midstream urinary (MSU) sample should be sent for microscopy and culture. Specific cultures may be required for tuberculosis or schistosomiasis. A random blood sugar level should be checked for diabetes. Baseline renal functions should be checked in a long-standing problem and with evidence of upper renal tract involvement.

An abdominal ultrasound and TVS should be performed to look for pelvic masses compressing urinary tract (ovarian cysts, big fibroids), bladder and ureteric diverticulae, post void urinary residual volume. Both kidneys and urinary tract should be visualized for pressure effects, hydronephrosis and calculi. Intravenous urogram may be required to visualize the anatomy in select cases. If no abnormality is detected urodynamics should be offered to allow detection of vesico-uretric reflux, urethral pressure profile and pressure flow studies.

Bladder cystoscopy and if required directed biopsy should be undertaken to rule out intravesical pathology like bladder calculi, diverticulae, polyps and cystitis.

Management should be directed towards treatment of underlying pathology. General advice on personal hygiene, regular voiding and adequate fluid intake should be given.

Specific antibiotics should be added after culture reports. Urinary culture should be repeated after 2 weeks to check the effectiveness of treatment. If no specific cause is identified, long-term low dose prophylactic antibiotics like norfloxacin, cephalosporin or trimethoprim should be added along with a urinary antiseptic.

3. **A mother brings her 8-year-old daughter to your clinic. She is anxious about the breast development in the child. How will you counsel her?**

Thelarche precedes the onset of adrenarche (development of axillary and pubic hair) and menarche (onset of menstruation) at the time of puberty. The average age of puberty is declining. Onset of puberty at 8 years of age is now considered normal. Hence, the mother should be counseled that this may be a normal sequence of events.

The child should be examined to see the Tanner staging of breast development and the presence of other signs of puberty like axillary and pubic hair. If there are no other signs of puberty then it could be a case of isolated thelarche. This usually arrests at Tanner stage 3. An X-ray of the wrist joint for bone age should be done and if corresponding to bone age, the child should be kept under follow-up for appearance of signs of puberty.

If thelarche is a part of growth spurt, adrenarche, menarche and presence of acne and body odor prior to completing 8 years of age, then she is a case of precocious puberty. Three quarter of cases of precocious puberty are idiopathic, however rare conditions like osteogenesis imperfecta, hypothalamic or pituitary lesions need to be ruled out.

Gn-RH agonists can be used to suppress the changes if they are causing psychological embarrassment. Depot monthly injections are used for 3-6 months. Longer use may predispose to osteoporosis.

4. Endometrial ablation is superior to hysterectomy. Debate.

With endometrial ablation, dysmenorrhea might not be relieved.

Pre-menstrual syndrome might not be relieved. Menstrual loss might remain unacceptable and might require further surgery. Subsequent surgery is contraindicated and the technique is more appropriate at the latter end of reproductive life. There is a range of different ablative techniques with different risks, efficacy and cost.

Endometrial ablation is effective in controlling dysfunctional uterine bleeding if there is no evidence of complex hyperplasia or malignancy on histopathological evaluation. It has the advantage of preserving the uterus, and preserving orgasmic sexual function in the young patient. Hysterectomy even with preservation of both ovaries leads to osteoporosis due to ovarian dysfunction. Endometrial ablation will prevent the development of osteoporosis premenopausally.

Endometrial ablation can be performed by thermal balloons, transcervical resection of endometrium (TCRE), microwave ablation.

Performance of endometrial ablation TCRE requires development of surgical skills which has a long learning curve. Reports of uterine perforation and injury to other abdominal organs with cautery has been reported. Absorption of large quantities of glycine leads to hyponatraemia, which can prove fatal if not treated promptly.

In comparison thermal balloon ablation and microwave ablation are relatively safer but complete amenorrhea may not be achieved in all patients and occasionally symptoms may return due to regeneration of endometrium. This may require repeat ablation or a hysterectomy. In the event of complex endometrial hyperplasia or endometrial cancer, there is no role for endometrial ablation and a hysterectomy is warranted.

Hence, the role of endometrial ablation is limited to benign conditions where expertise and/or equipment exists for performance of endometrial ablation. However, recurrence of symptoms and a higher rate of complications restricts its use. Otherwise it is certainly superior to hysterectomy.

PAPER 9

1. **Discuss the morbidity of chemotherapeutic agents used for treatment of ovarian cancer and measures that might be taken to minimize them.**

Note: The morbidity should be for general chemotherapeutic agents and specific to the treatment protocols. Similarly, preventive steps can be dealt into separate categories—general and specific.

All the relevant baseline tests should be performed, e.g. Full blood counts, renal function, and ECG and patient fully assessed prior to chemotherapy.

The possible side effects include nausea and vomiting, bone marrow suppression, infection, and leukemia.

Cisplatin and carboplatin are the most effective agents for management of ovarian cancer. Carboplatin is being increasingly used as it is better tolerated and has an equivalent efficacy. Carboplatin and Paclitaxel combination is considered standard treatment now.

Paclitaxel: Alkylating agents have a radiomimitic action and act or rapidly dividing cells of bone marrow and GIT. Agranulocytosis and aplastic anemia along with GI complications have high incidence.

Toxicity can be assessed by monitoring FBC and differential white cell count and platelets, renal and liver function tests.

The measures to minimize side effects are:

Sedation, effective anti-emetics prior to and during treatment, steroids and H_2 antagonists.

Adequate fluid loading prior to commensing chemotherapeutic agents of cytotoxic agents should be administered slowly.

Limitation of treatment if no response after three pulses of therapy.

Limitation of treatment to one year beyond which it is not helpful and risk of leukemia is increased.

Alopecia is prevented by selection of appropriate chemotherapy, other methods of prevention are not of proven efficacy.

Specialised support and treatment in a cancer centre. Support group based counseling is helpful while the patient is hospitalized.

2. **A 22-year-old woman presents at your clinic complaining of foul smelling discharge. She had a normal vaginal delivery one week back in your hospital. On examination you found a retained swab in her vagina. She is furious at the development and threatens to sue the hospital. Outline your further course of action.**

Senior obstetric team member should preferably counsel this patient. The retained swab should be removed and a high vaginal swab should be taken for culture and sensitivity. Her vital signs such as pulse, blood pressure and temperature should be checked. Complete blood count should be checked to assess her white cell count. There is a possibility of gram-negative and anaerobic septicaemia which can present with low blood pressure, tachycardia or high temperature. If symptomatic she should be covered with appropriate antibiotics for gram-negative and anaerobic organisms like a combination of metronidazole with third generation cephalosporin or quinolones.

She should be patiently counseled that her symptoms had resulted from a retained swab. She should be informed that it is a rare occurrence and since it has been removed now it will not lead to any further complications. She should also be explained that to prevent such an occurrence the swabs are counted by the nurse/midwife prior to and after any surgical procedure. Occasionally there may be an error in counting which can result in this condition.

Empathy and apology should be offered on behalf of the hospital. If she still wishes to sue the hospital she should be supplied with the necessary forms and procedural documents.

A follow-up visit should be arranged for checking the HVS result, and prescribing appropriate antibiotics and to dispel any further doubts.

3. A 15-year-old sexually active woman comes to you for contraceptive advice. How will you counsel her?

Establish a good rapport with her by being gentle, objective and non-judgmental. Identify the reason for this visit, and other sexual and mental health issues involved. Discuss the emotional and physical implications of sexual activity, including the risks of pregnancy and sexually transmitted infections.

Assess her competence to consent to treatment by her ability to understand the information provided, to weigh up the risks and benefits, and to express her own wishes.

Elicit her education status, social and financial support, previous sexual, menstrual and reproductive history along with alcohol, cigarette and drug abuse.

If she is assessed competent, proper documentation of her being 'Fraser ruling competent' (that she understands the advice, will have or continue to have sex, she has been advised to inform her parents, this is in her best interest) should be made in her case notes.

Acknowledge her right to confidentiality from healthcare professionals and provide information leaflets mentioning the risks and benefits of various contraceptive choices, sexual health and other lifestyle issues, and appropriate website addresses. Make her aware of the law in relation of sexual activity with a young person and that her consent would be sought if information is to be shared or confidentiality breached. However, consent is not essential if the disclosure is justified.

She may use combined oral contraceptives (COC), the progestogen only pill (POP), and the progestogen only implant and injections. All medical contraindications should be ruled out and general advise regarding the risks and benefits of individual methods should be imparted to her. Give her time and support to make an informed choice. Use of condoms and safe sex practices should be promoted at all times for prevention of STIs and HIV.

The effect of hormonal contraception on Bone mineral density is superceded by the effect of factors like exercise, nutrition, calcium intake, and smoking.

Explore the possibility of exploitation and abuse by enquiring whether the relationship is mutually agreed. Child protection agencies should be contacted on suspicion.

Whether she wants to inform her GP. Encourage discussion with a parent, carer or another trusted adult. Respect any refusal.

Assess any additional counseling or support needs. Arrange appropriate follow-up after 3 months or whenever they develop any problems with the contraception.

Note: The legal age of consent to sexual activity in Scotland, England and Wales is 16 years. Sexual activity under the age of 16 years is an offence even if consensual or both parties are aged under 16 years. The offence is committed by the person who has sexual intercourse or other sexual activity with the person under 16 years – not by the person aged under 16 herself.

The legal guidance issued in 1986 after the Gillick case states that health care professionals are justified in giving confidential contraceptive advice and treatment to under 16s provided that **(Gillick's Competence)**—

She/he understands the advice provided and its implications.

Her/his mental or physical health would otherwise be likely to suffer and so provision of advice or treatment is in their best interest.

When it is believed that there is a risk to the health, safety or welfare of a young person or others which is so serious as to outweigh the young person's right to privacy, they should follow agreed child protection protocols.

FRASER guidelines issued in 1985 during the Gillick's case hearing are—

The young person understands the health professional's advice;

The health professional cannot persuade the young person to inform his/her parent or allow the doctor to inform the parents that he/she is seeking contraceptive advice;

The young person is very likely to begin or continue having intercourse with or without contraceptive treatment.

Unless he or she receives contraceptive advice or treatment, the young person's physical or mental health or both are likely to suffer.

The young person's best interests require the health professional to give contraceptive advice, treatment or both without parental consent.

SEXUAL offences Act 2003 states that

A person is not guilty of aiding, abetting or counseling a sexual offence against a child where they are acting for the purpose of:

• Protecting a child from pregnancy or sexually transmitted infection,
• Protecting the physical safety of a child,
• Promoting a child's emotional well-being by the giving of advice.

Over 25% of young people aged under16 are sexually active but as a group are least likely to use contraception including condoms.

Three out of 4 parents with a child under 18 feel that young people should have access to confidential contraceptive advice (BMRB survey 2004).

Provision of such services does not lead to earlier sexual activity.

4. Discuss the changing role of HRT in the treatment of menopausal symptoms after WHI (Women's Health Initiative) study.

Till recently, before the results of WHI were published, the estrogen component of HRT was used to prevent hot flushes, night sweats, vaginal dryness, depression, loss of energy and libido. The progesterone component protected the endometrium from estrogenic effects. The long-term benefits were thought to be protection from osteoporosis, reduction in colon cancer, coronary artery disease and prevention of heart attacks. The downside was a possible slight increase in breast cancer which was countered by studies showing an increased survival in these women.

The WHI study along with Million Women Study (MWS) reported that estrogens increased the rates of heart attacks, strokes, venous thrombo-embolism and breast cancer in women taking HRT. The estrogen—only arm of the WHI was stopped prematurely in March 2004 due to an extra number of strokes in the study group. It also reported that the quality of life was not improved with HRT. Following this, in Dec 2003, the UK CSM advised that HRT should no longer be the first choice for the prevention and treatment of osteoporosis.

There have been concerns about the flaws in the study design of WHI and MWS. When the estrogen arm of WHI study was stopped, it did not report any increase in breast cancer or heart attacks even after 7 years of treatment which has created confusion over the actual implication of HRT.

WHI reported a slight increase in coronary heart disease in the first year of use but not in subsequent years confirming that estrogens commenced in older women of 60-79 years may do early harm in the form of heart attacks, strokes and vascular dementia before any benefit is achieved. Oestrogens appear to have no place for the secondary prevention of cardiovascular disease. There is also an increased risk of venous thromboembolism, and breast cancer with the combined hormonal preparations. On the contrary if a younger population from 50-59 is examined, HRT leads to over forty percent decrease in heart attacks and colorectal cancers, and more than 25 percent decrease in breast cancer and overall mortality.

Currently proven benefits of HRT are an improvement of symptoms such as hot flushes, night sweats, insomnia, vaginal dryness, and peri-menopausal depression and also a decrease in colon cancer, vertebral and hip fractures. The dose and route of administration will depend upon the symptoms, and the age of the patient. Peri-menopausal and post-menopausal patients with vasomotor symptoms should be given either oral or transdermal oestradiol with cyclical progestogen in the lowest effective dose; for the shortest duration (five years). Women on HRT with combined preparations or on estrogens alone are recommended to have a yearly review of symptoms and mammogram along with 6 monthly breast examination.

PAPER 10

1. Teenage pregnancy is a social problem. Discuss the steps that need to be taken to reduce this burden.

The UK has the highest number of under 18 and under 16 conception rates in western Europe. Though the incidence is reducing over the years, it still contributes significantly to poverty, inequality and poor aspirations in those involved. Department of health (DOH) launched 'Teenage Pregnancy Strategy" in 1999 which has resulted in an all time low teenage pregnancy rates. The target is to halve the existing rates by 2010.

There is significant variation in the pregnancy rates in various locations. The problem should be given equal priority in all areas so its uptake is encouraged.

There is a strong link of higher teenage pregnancy rates to deprived population, in particular those having poor educational attainment and low aspiration. The short- and long-term consequences of early parenthood in terms of poorer health and education outcomes for teenage mothers and their children should be highlighted at every given opportunity. Parents should be encouraged to talk to their teens about sex issues openly.

To reduce teenage pregnancies, there should be active engagement of all the key mainstream delivery partners—Health, education, social services and youth support services—and the voluntary sector. A locally active senior person should be accountable for, and leading the local strategy.

A well publicized, young people centered contraceptive and sexual advice service should be easily available. All schools should have comprehensive teaching programmes on sex and relationship education, which should be given high priority in the school curriculum.

Adopt a targeted approach on 'At risk' population, specially the deprived and looked after children. Children born to teenage parents are more likely, in time to become teenage parents themselves. Young people should be kept motivated to pursue further learning or a career, rather than to choose or accept early parenthood.

2. You are the SpR on emergency duty and have just received information that the duty SHO has perforated the uterus while performing MTP. Enumerate your initial assessment, management and the course of action in the postpartum period.

Reach the operation theater and inform the anaesthetist about the perforation if it has not been done so far. Instruct the theater nurse to prepare for laparoscopy and a possible laparotomy. Elicit a brief history from SHO or nurse about the patient, her gestational age, the uterine size, whether it was a anomalous uterus, which instrument perforated the uterus and the approximate blood loss. All this should preferably be done while scrubbing.

Enquire about the vital parameters of the patient from anaesthetist. Tell him to proceed with resuscitation and intubation of the patient. Another large bore 14G cannula needs to be inserted for appropriate fluid replacement and blood samples withdrawn for urgent hemoglobin, cross match and clotting studies. Theater nurse should be instructed to insert a Foley's catheter to moniter the urinary output.

A per speculum examination should be done to determine the amount of bleeding through the os. A per vaginal examination should be performed to ascertain the uterine size. Two or more units of blood should be ordered and constant vigil on vital should be maintained.

A diagnostic laparoscopy should be performed to assess the damage to uterus, bladder and bowel. MTP should be completed under direct vision.

If the perforation is small with no visible injury elsewhere and no active bleeding, patient is managed expectantly. Antibiotics and oxytocics should be administered.

If the perforation is bleeding actively and is not controlled by pressure, laparotomy is required. Senior anaesthetist and Gynecology consultant should be called for. Hemostatic sutures need to be applied and bladder and bowel inspected for possible damage. If in doubt, a general surgeon should be called for help.

A large profusely bleeding perforation may on occasion require a hysterectomy for hemostasis. This decision should be taken by the senior most gynaecologist present. Postoperative antibiotics and adequate Thromboprophylaxis should be given.

Postoperatively, all the notes should be meticulously completed with detailed operation notes. Risk management forms should be filled and the situation explained to the patient at the first opportune moment when she is comfortable. All her queries should be answered clearly and if the situation demands contraception should be discussed. Patient's consultant and GP should be informed about the incident and follow-up visit arranged prior to discharge.

3. **A 36-year-old woman has been referred to you by the GP. She is anxious on account of the death of her mother due to metastatic ovarian cancer and is worried that she may die of the same. Her elder sister is on treatment with Tamoxifen for breast cancer. How will you counsel her?**

It is known that women with a first degree relative with breast cancer have a two-fold risk of development of breast cancer compared to the normal population. Two first degree relatives increase this risk to four-fold. This has been traced to genetic inheritance. In the past decade it has been observed that an abnormality in the BRCA -1 gene increases susceptibility to both breast and ovarian cancer. This gene is localized to the long arm of chromosome 17 and is transmitted by autosomal dominant inheritance. Over half the women who inherit this gene from either the mother or the father will develop breast cancer by 50 years of age. The lifetime risk of breast cancer in such patients is 80%.

Similarly the lifetime risk of ovarian cancer in the general population is 1 in 70. If a first degree relative has ovarian cancer the risk is 5% and if two first degree relatives have it the risk is 7%. The hereditary syndromes described are a site specific ovarian cancer syndrome and breast ovarian cancer syndrome.

A second gene BRCA-2 gene is located on chromosome 13. Its presence confers a high risk for early development of breast cancer but is not associated with ovarian cancer.

Hence this woman can be offered screening for both breast and ovarian cancers. Her options are to have breast screening with regular monthly self-breast examination and yearly mammography. Ovarian screening is done by yearly pelvic examination, trans-vaginal ultrasound coupled with color Doppler and CA 125 levels.

She should be counseled that she can undergo screening for mutated BRCA 1 and 2 genes. If negative it will be reassuring. However, if positive, it may warrant prophylactic oophorectomy and even prophylactic mastectomy. The decision to undertake this test must be made by the patient depending on her psychological concern.

4. **A 15-year-old girl comes to your clinic accompanied by her mother and reveals that she has not started to menstruate yet. Outline the briefs of your history, examination and investigations.**

The commonest cause of primary amenorrhea is constitutional delay. A history of delayed menarche or polycystic ovarian syndrome (PCO) in mother or sisters is relevant and may suggest a similar trend in the girl. Past history of any prolonged illness, trauma to skull, radiotherapy, chemotherapy, or medications like steroids or anti-hypertensives that may have interfered with pituitary function, should be enquired. It is important to enquire about features suggestive of intracranial lesions, like headaches, and visual field defects.

The order and age of development of breasts, axillary and pubic hair should be enquired to determine her development phase. Excessive sporting activity and recent weight loss may cause hypothalamic amenorrhea.

She should be taken into confidence and enquiry made into family or school stresses, parental expectations and self image. This is best achieved in the absence of mother in the room. History of substance abuse and drugs should be gently elicited.

During her examination, the height, weight and body mass index (BMI) should be calculated. Secondary sexual characteristics should be examined to note her Tanner's staging. Short height, with widely spaced nipples, wide carrying angle and webbed neck may suggest Turner's syndrome. Appropriate height with evidence of obesity, acne and hirsutism suggest PCO. A tall girl with good breast development and scanty pubic hair could indicate androgen insensitivity. Galactorrhoea and thyroid enlargement should be looked for.

Inspection of external genitalia should be done to exclude an imperforate hymen. A per vaginal examination is not indicated.

The investigations and further management are guided by her history. In constitutional delays the option of not doing anything should be offered to the woman.

Karyotyping may reveal Turner's syndrome (45 X) or androgen insensitivity (46 XY). Pituitary gonadatotropins; follicle stimulating hormone (FSH) and Leutinising hormone (LH) should be measured. Raised levels are suggestive of primary gonadal dysgenesis, and low levels indicate hypothalamic hypogonadism. A raised LH/FSH ratio suggests PCO.

Thyroid stimulating hormone (TSH), serum prolactin, testosterone, 17-beta-estradiol and sex hormone binding globulin (SHBG) should be advised if indicated by history. An abdominal ultrasound should be performed to confirm the presence of uterus and upper vagina. It will also help to rule out cryptomenorrhea.

Note: *Failure of development of secondary sexual characteristics by age 14 and failure to menstruate by 16 years, in the presence of secondary sexual characters, should be investigated.*

PAPER 11

1. Discuss the ethical issues involved with human cloning.

Cloning involves having multiple, exactly similar genetic copies of the original organism. Human cloning involves creation of an embryo by extracting DNA from specialized non-sexual cells, and subsequent implantation into an egg whose DNA nucleus has been removed.

Proponents of cloning suggest that it might serve as an efficacious treatment for infertility, enabling people to pass their genes to future generations. Early human experiments, however, are likely to result in a number of clinical failures and lead to miscarriage, necessitating hundreds of abortions, or births of massively deformed offsprings. A number of such defects may not manifest themselves till a clone is mature, leading to its death.

There are ethical concerns about the first clone and the issues that will arise should cloning succeed in producing a healthy child. A cloned embryo does not qualify to be the same as a conceived embryo as it logically does not have a set of parents and the parent actually is genetically its monozygotic twin. There are concerns about how such clones will relate to other kind of families and accept their social and parental responsibilities.

Legal experts argue that cloning may violate, for example, a child's right to an open future. A child born as a genetic copy of another may feel undue pressure to become like or different from its progenitor. But this possibility exists even for children born to normal parents.

Are we trying to play God by "making" babies rather than "having them"? Will the society accept procedure failures' deformed offsprings? "Who is socially responsible for them? Will they have rights and legal protection? Are we justified in interfering with nature?" Are some of the questions that need to be answered.

Note: Any ethical question needs to be divided into 4 principles:
Respect for Autonomy, Beneficience, Non-malpractice and Justice.

2. A 75-year-old woman was clinically diagnosed with lichen sclerosis. Discuss her management.

Lichen sclerosis causes intense pruritis vulvae. It is important to note that vulval carcinoma can occur in 3-5% patients of lichen sclerosis. Besides squamous hyperplasia or vulval intraepithelial neoplasia (VIN) has been seen in biopsy specimens adjacent to lichen sclerosis in half the patients. Hence, a biopsy of the lesion is warranted especially if there is a doubt over the diagnosis, or there are suspicious areas or there has been a failure of medical treatment.

Since the etiology is thought to be autoimmune, treatment is with topical steroid cream application. However, milder steroid creams like 1% hydrocortisone may not provide relief of symptoms. It is then justified to use stronger steroid creams like clobetasol (Dermovate), betamethasone or fluocinalone. These can be applied every night during an acute episode and then two to three times a week during remission.

During periods of remission weaker steroid creams like hydrocortisone may also be used daily. Some patients may be controlled on emollients alone during remission.

Use of estrogen creams is of no value as there are no estrogen receptors on the vulval skin.

Testosterone creams have been used with good relief of symptoms. However, the testosterone gets absorbed and may cause hirsutism. Others feel that testosterone only exerts a placebo effect.

Local destructive procedures like cryo-cautery or CO_2 laser have no role as they only remove the epidermis and do not treat the underlying changes within the dermis. Healing may be prolonged and may produce more discomfort and distortion.

Simple vulvectomy cannot be justified in lichen sclerosis as it often recurs in the excision margins. However, it is justified if hyperkeratotic patches appear or there is a suspicion of malignancy.

3. A 52-year-old postmenopausal woman complains of hot flushes. She is on treatment with Tamoxifen for breast cancer and wishes to start HRT. How will you counsel her?

HRT is effective for symptomatic relief of menopausal symptoms and its use is justified if symptoms are adversely affecting her quality of life. However, she should be made aware of the risks and allowed to make an informed choice.

Details of her complaint, its effect on her quality of life, duration of menopause (prophylactic oophorectomy?), expectations from treatment along with family and treatment history should be enquired for a need and risk analysis.

Recent bone densitometry, baseline LFT, RFT, should be advised. If possible the oncologist supervising the women's treatment should be consulted regarding the status of her cancer.

For mildly symptomatic women, lifestyle changes (limit smoking, alcohol, and caffeine and start moderate weight bearing exercises) combined with non-prescription medications like dietary isoflavones, mineral and calcium supplements and vitamin E may be prescribed. Safety of black cohosh is not proven in women taking tamoxifen. She should avoid known triggers for vasomotor symptoms like hot and spicy foods or drinks, hot environment and stress. Weight gain should be kept under check.

HRT increases the risk of breast cancer and is related to the duration of therapy. Therapy with combined estrogens and progestogens is contraindicated in women with breast cancer.

Tibolone is effective in the treatment of hot flushes and may also increase the risk of breast cancer but lesser than the risk by combined hormonal preparations.

Progestogens such as norethisterone 5 mg/day or megestrol acetate 40 mg/day are effective in control of hot flushes but may flare progesterone receptor positive breast cancer.

Selective serotonin reuptake inhibitors (SSRIs) may be helpful in treating hot flushes and are not contraindicated in breast cancer. Its use may be associated with temporary decrease in libido.

Multidisciplinary counseling should be encouraged. Prior to commencement of treatment she should discuss its effect on her condition with her Oncologist. Contact numbers of local support groups of menopausal women should be provided.

Information leaflets documenting risks and benefits of individual HRT preparations should be provided and follow-up appointment in the menopausal clinic arranged.

4. Debate on the prospects of prophylactic HPV vaccines.

A question on debate must include pros and cons of the subject.

Prophylactic vaccines prevent the initial HPV infection in the genital tract and thus prevent the subsequent development of anogenital neoplasia. This will bring down the associated mortality and morbidity.

Current vaccines are directed against high risk HPV 16 and 18 types (type specific) and thus cannot confer protection against anogenital carcinoma by other low risk HPV like types 6 and 11.

Majority of sexually active women acquire ($\geq$ 70% lifetime risk) an HPV infection at some time in their lifetime. Target population is difficult to identify. Vaccination of adolescent girls before they commence sexual activity is proposed but is difficult due to variable coitarche.

Vaccination of all men may be effective but is not cost effective and acceptability is questionable.

Vaccine delivery to target population may be difficult as it involves vaccinating young adults 3 times over 6 months period. School health services may need to be involved.

Public acceptability of vaccine may vary according to the education and social levels. General reluctance to discuss sexual issues and social stigma may hinder acceptance of vaccination against asexually transmitted disease. Public education to dispel misdirected fears will be required.

Vaccination can lead to false sense of security in the minds of women and can decrease the cervical screening uptake. This may paradoxically increase the incidence of cervical cancer.

Current vaccines are expensive to manufacture and maintain. Cost will be a concern especially for low resource settings till cheaper, single dose vaccines are made available.

Note: Future II study is currently underway in which women 16-23 years received 3 doses of quadrivalent vaccine. 2 years postvaccination follow-up has revealed 100% efficacy.

PAPER 12

1. What precautions and preventive steps can be taken to minimize adhesion formation following gynecological surgery?

Careful patient selection along with the skill and experience of surgeon should be optimum for any surgery. Women undergoing high risk surgeries should be informed of the risk of adhesions and adhesion reduction strategies should also be discussed with them as part of risk management.

For the majority of women, adhesions do not appear to have any particular consequences.

Laparoscopic surgery is associated with much less adhesion formation and its use should be preferred over conventional surgery wherever possible. If the level of skill is not present then the women should be referred to a tertiary center.

Principles of microsurgery should be adopted with careful tissue handling, copious irrigation to avoid tissue desiccation and meticulous attention to hemostasis. Intraperitoneal infection should be avoided and contamination with foreign particles like glove powder minimized. Fine non-reactive suture material should be used and excessive cauterization avoided, preventing tissue ischemia.

Physical adhesion barriers like Interceed can decrease adhesion formation if hemostasis is meticulous. Seprafilm sheets, surgiwrap and spraygel are available but are site specific.

Iso-osmotic solutions like Hartmann's solution, Hyskon, icodextrin and Adept may cause large reduction in non-surgical site adhesions. It has been one of the primary methods to decrease adhesions, is easy to use and also minimizes capillary oozing.

Note: SCAR study was done to determine the impact of adhesions on gynecologic surgery. Ovary was found to be the most adhesiogenic organ in pelvic surgery and myomectomy, most adhesiogenic gynae surgery. Fibrin deposition is the first step in adhesion formation and usually starts within 3 hours of surgery. It is reversible in the initial phases.

2. **An 18-year-old presents at the Accident and Emergency. She is terrified and anxious and reveals that she has been sexually assaulted by her boy friend. She does not wish to involve the police yet. You are the Ob/Gyn registrar on emergency duty.**

a. **What relevant facts should be kept in mind before you examine her?**

As a competent adult she has a choice as to whether to involve the police. She should be put at ease and her dignity should be maintained at all times. She should be informed that she has a right to refuse any part of examination.

Any information provided about the assault should be recorded and kept separately from the clinical notes. The women should be shown these notes and informed that in case she changes her mind later on and wants to involve the police, this information can be utilized.

b. **How will you examine and investigate her?**

Offer her a complete general medical examination. Document any injuries, marks or stains and provide first aid for minor injuries. Vulval hair clipping, vaginal/oral/anal swabs should be taken according to local protocols, labeled and stored in appropriate medium for a possible later use. Endocervical swabs should be taken for sexually transmitted infections. Investigation and treatment of more serious injuries should be promptly undertaken.

c. **How will you manage her condition?**

She should be encouraged to talk to a supportive friend or a family member. Replacement underclothing should be arranged and the clothes worn at the time of assault bagged. Safe accommodation on discharge should be discussed with her.

Emergency contraception with levonorgestrel 1.5 mg within 72 hours or copper intrauterine device within 5 days should be discussed and appropriate choices offered.

With the woman's consent her GP should be appraised. Adequate follow-up should be organized in relation to emergency contraception, STI testing and counseling.

If her assailant has obvious risk factors for HBV or HIV, urgent advice should be sought from genitourinary physician and post exposure prophylaxis against sexually transmitted infections (Hepatitis B, HIV) administered. If post exposure prophylaxis has not been given, she should be referred to GUM clinic after 14 days for an STI screen.

If the woman refuses to give written consent for police involvement, the samples must be destroyed.

Note: Hepatitis B prophylaxis should commence as early as possible after exposure and within 72 hours.

3. **A 28-year-old woman complains of persistent vaginal discharge despite various medications given to her by the GP.**

a. **What can be the cause of her condition?**

Common causes of vaginal discharge in women of reproductive age group are physiological, infective (bacterial vaginosis, candidiasis, trichomoniasis, *Chlamydia trachomatis* and *Neisseria gonorrheae*), foreign bodies (forgotten tampons, condoms), cervical polyp and Ectropion, allergy and vary rarely genital tract malignancy.

b. **What will you look for during the initial assessment?**

Colour, amount, duration, consistency, associated smell or itch and the relation of discharge to menstrual cycle should be enquired. Any recent change in the nature of discharge or sexual partner should be noted. History of dysuria, dyspareunia, abdominal pain, fever, and abnormal bleeding pattern should be asked.

Enquire about sexual and contraceptive history, menstrual history (pregnancy, post abortion or postpartum), associated medical conditions (diabetes) and medications (antibiotics, corticosteroids) along with previous treatment history. Compliance with previous medication and side effects like vomiting should be checked.

Assess her risk for sexually transmitted infections (STI). Even in the absence of other factors, recurrent infection refractory to treatment requires laboratory investigations.

Palpate abdomen for any pain, inspect vulva for any obvious discharge and vulvitis.

A gentle per speculum examination should be done after cleaning the vulva with saline (avoid antiseptics). Inspect vaginal walls, cervix, foreign bodies and nature of discharge. High vaginal and endocervical swabs should be taken at this time. Test vaginal pH from lateral vaginal walls using narrow range pH paper.

Perform a bimanual pelvic examination for cervical motion tenderness, uterine and adnexal tenderness. High vaginal swab should be sent for:

- Microscopy and Gram stain for diagnosis of BV (Amsel's criteria) and Candida spores.
- Saline wet microscopy for diagnosis of Trichomonas vaginalis (direct visualization).
- Culture in chocolate agar for diagnosis of *Neisseria gonorrhoeae* (Sabouraud's medium for Candida if microscopy is inconclusive).
- Sensitivities: to various locally available treatment regimens.

Endocervical swab should be sent for culture, ELISA, and NAAT for *N. gonnorhoeae* and *C. trachomatis*.

c. What advice will you give regarding her condition?

Provide appropriate treatment with locally available protocols. Metronidazole and clotrimazole are usually the first line treatment. For recurrent infection, a weakly dose can be continued for 6 months.

She should avoid douching, local irritants, perfumed products, tight fitting synthetic clothing. Avoid alcohol intake with metronidazole.

If diagnosis is STI, partner notification and treatment, referral to GUM clinic and specialist advice should be sought. Routine screening and treatment of male partners is not required.

Barrier contraceptives may get damaged with vaginal preparations containing clotrimazole. Abstinence or double protection should be advised.

Note: Commonest cause of vaginal discharge in young women is physiological. Commonest infective cause is bacterial vaginosis (not considered a sexually transmitted disease but is associated with early sexual activity and higher number of sexual partners), followed by candidiasis. Commonest bacterial STI is *C. trachomatis*.

Risk factors to be sought for STI are: age ≤ 25 years, change in sexual partner in the last year; more than one sexual partner in the last year.

If High vaginal swab cannot be transported immediately to the laboratory, it should be stored at 4 degrees C for less than 48 hours.

ELISA—Enzyme-linked immunosorbent assay.

NAAT—Nucleic acid amplification tests.

BV—Bacterial vaginosis.

Incubation period (days) of various STIs are:

Neisseria gonorrheae	2-7
Herpes simplex virus	2-12
Trichomonas vaginalis	4-20
Chlamydia trachomatis	7-14
Treponema pallidum	14-84
Human immunodeficiency virus	30-90
Human papilloma virus (HPV)	30-140
Hepatitis B virus	45-180

4. **A young woman presents at the Accident and Emergency complaining of severe abdominal pain and bloating. She has been on injection Menogon for the treatment of infertility. Her last period was 20 days back.**

a. **What investigations relevant to her condition will you order?**

The most likely diagnosis is Ovarian Hyperstimulation syndrome. Investigations should include FBC, hematocrit, urea and electrolytes, creatinine, liver function test, coagulation profile, ultrasound scanning, chest X-ray and serum pregnancy test.

b. **How will you manage her condition?**

She should be admitted in the hospital and investigated to establish the severity of her condition, preferably under the supervision of a specialist in reproductive medicine. Multidisciplinary team input may be required for patient care.

Hypovolaemia should be corrected by infusion of Hartmann's solution or normal saline, with added potassium if required. Use of albumin solution is controversial. The use of plasma expanders like hydroxyethyl starch is better than hemaccel which gives a temporary relief.

Thromboprophylaxis with heparin is necessary. Mannitol or dopamine may be required in oliguric patients. Prostaglandin synthetase inhibitors should be avoided for analgesia as they may decrease the renal blood flow.

Close monitoring of pulse, respiratory rate, blood pressure, temperature, fluid balance and urinary output should be maintained. Hematological parameters and abdominal girth measurements should be repeated every day initially. An in-dwelling catheter may be required, if the output is low/ difficult to measure or in the presence of voiding difficulties. Additional monitoring with pulse oxymetry or admission to intensive care unit will depend on the severity of the condition.

Drainage of third space accumulations may be necessary to improve distress and urinary output. Abdominal or pleural paracentesis should be done under ultrasound guidance.

Surgical intervention should preferably be avoided but may be required in cases of ovarian torsion or significant intraperitoneal bleeding.

Note: A hematocrit greater than 0.44 or abnormal liver or renal functions indicate a need for hospitalization.

Index